FULL-BODY FITNESS FOR RUNNERS

FOR RUNNERS

Run Longer, Stronger, Faster

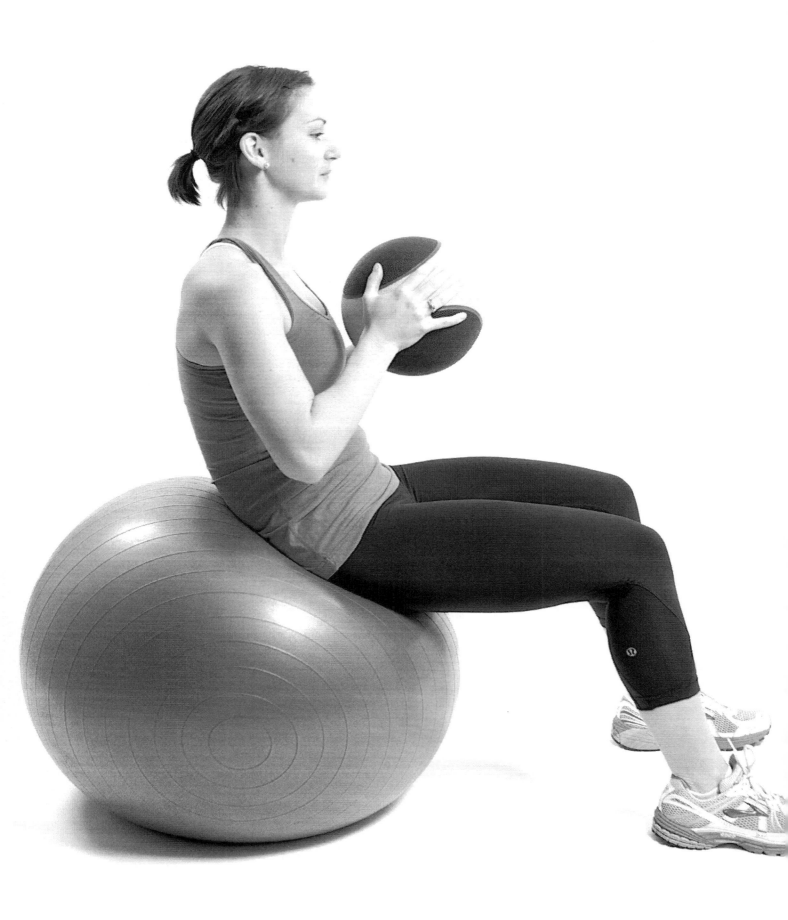

FULL-BODY FITNESS FOR RUNNERS
Run Stronger, Longer, Faster

Written by Thad H. McLaurin

Foreword by Jef Mallett

Contributors:

Jeff Galloway

Dean Karnazes

Sage Rountree

Danny Dreyer

Kate Percy

Troy Busot

Robin Thurston

Toby Guillette

Judy Staveley

Ben Greenfield

Kenny Santucci

Chef Brandon McDearis

Jason Robillard

Chef Stefan Czapalay

Kevin Leathers

Laura Buxenbaum

Edited by

Iris Sutcliffe

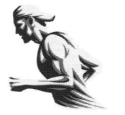

RunnerDude's Fitness

2014

First Printing: 2014

ISBN 978-0-692-02695-3

RunnerDude's Fitness
2309 W. Cone Blvd., Ste. 120
Greensboro, NC 27408

www.runnerdudesfitness.com

Dedication

To my parents and my immediate family—Mitzi, Duncan, Rayna, and Ellery—and to my extended running family.

Thank you.

Without your support and patience, I would have never achieved my dream of opening RunnerDude's Fitness and writing this book.

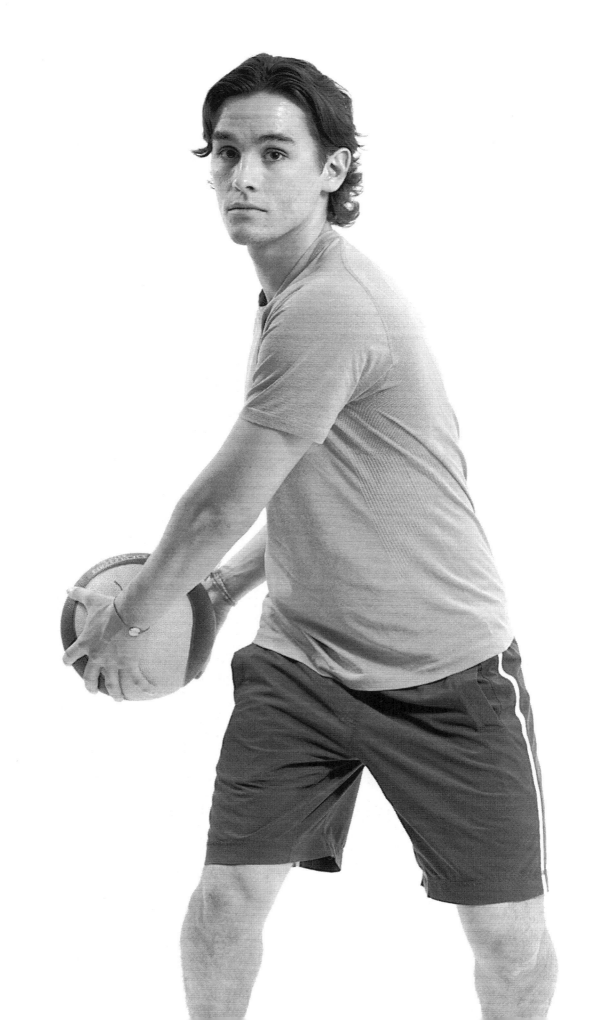

Contents

Acknowledgments

I want to thank every runner I've ever run with and every client I've ever trained. You've taught me more about coaching and running than I'll ever learn in a class. Every runner I work with is a new experience. No two runners are the same. That's what's fun about coaching. It's always new. I'm always learning. Thanks.

Thanks also to Alan Wiest, my instructor at the National Personal Training Institute. You gave me the foundation for understanding how the body works inside and out. This has made me a better trainer and coach. Thanks.

Special thanks to clients and friends Matthew Halip and Kristen Bowles for graciously agreeing to model the exercises in this book. You gave up an entire day for posing, posing, and more posing. You did a great job. Thanks.

Huge thanks to all the contributors to the book, in particular to Jef Mallett for providing the foreword, awesome original illustration, and ongoing support; Iris Sutcliffe for her editorial wisdom and guidance; and to Jeff Galloway for taking the time to share his running nutrition wisdom. Thanks.

Photographic Credits

Exercise and Back Cover Photography: Daniel Rice, Allez Photography

Front Cover Photography, page 11: Deno Kontoulas, 48 Layers Photography

Other Photography: CanStockPhoto.com or as noted by photo credit

Photographic Editing:
Daniel Rice
April McLaurin
Deno Kontoulas

Illustration (page 9): Jef Mallett

Exercise Models:
Kristen Bowles
Matthew Halip

Foreword

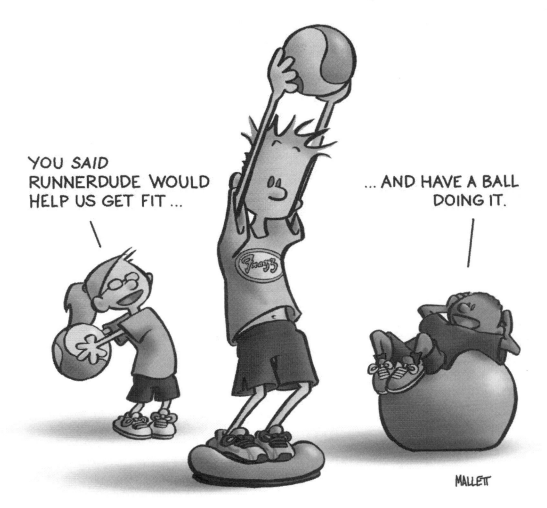

"You run?" That's a common question that people who aren't like us ask people who are. "For fun? Boy, you've got a weird hobby."

I am passionate about running, and I can accept its perceived weirdness as long as I don't have to defend it. It's not that running is indefensible. It's just that the details can be tough to convey. As the great trumpeter Dizzy Gillespie said about jazz: If you don't already understand, I can't explain it.

That's an embarrassing confession for me to make, because I write for a living. I should be able to explain anything I know and fake my way through what I don't. Then again, maybe not. I write fiction. Short stories. Very short stories; 365 of them every year.

I write and draw a comic strip. I'm passionate about that, too, but I'm no better at explaining how to do it. People ask very good questions: "Where do you get your ideas?" "Which is more important—drawing or writing?" "How do I get a job like that?"

I swear I don't know. I do it like I run. I just go out and do and try and sweat and bleed and create. I enjoy the flow when things do flow, and I try to remain calm and find a way through when things jam up. Also, like with running, I pay close attention to people who do it well, and then I try like mad to keep up.

That's why I pay a lot of attention to Thad the RunnerDude. Thad is a writer who can explain running. Maybe there's a runner out there who can explain writing the way Thad writes about running, but I think I'll go back to Dizzy Gillespie, or at least to jazz.

Writing, like running, like music, is a sometimes smooth, sometimes spastic, sometimes tedious process of collecting and arranging a bunch of wildly disparate elements until, if you do it right, they line up into a single moment of clarity.

I've had that moment. I've had a lot of those moments. Some of them have been profound, even life changing, but those are rare, and that's probably a good thing. Shaking up your life, even for the better, is exhausting work. I like small moments and lots of them. They can come from anywhere. They're not always recognizable at the time. They don't all come from running or sports or physical activity. Or any activity at all. A good book or sunrise will do most of the work for you. Some moments leave you thinking that every crappy day you've ever had, and every crappy day you'll have from here forward, was worth this moment. Some of them only have to be worth getting up in the morning. Just to complicate things, some of them might in fact include *not* getting up in the morning.

But I digress. I should get to my own moment before you wander off. And that's just it: None of those moments exist if you quit before you get to it. Runners know better than anybody about living in the moment, and that the process itself can be the reward, the journey can be the destination.

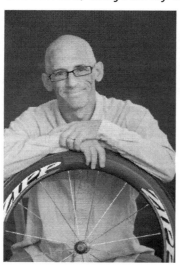

Just like a run is more than transportation, *Full-Body Fitness for Runners* is more than just information. Or entertainment, or inspiration. Or, come to that, only for runners. It's all of those, all lined up. It's what you came here for.

So take a moment and check out RunnerDude. Take several moments. He's got tons of 'em. He may step out for a run, but he'll never run out.

Jef Mallett is the author, illustrator, and creator of the nationally syndicated comic *Frazz* and author of *Trizophrenia: Inside the Minds of a Triathlete.*

Photo: Dave Trumpie

Preface

"Stand up straight." "Don't slouch." "Sit up." As a teenager, those were constant reminders from my parents and teachers. Of course at 15 I knew everything and shrugged off the comments as nagging. Plus, it actually felt uncomfortable to stand up straight.

Turns out, they were right. I was a *sloucher*. It wasn't until several years later, when I saw a profile picture of me, that I realized I actually did have bad posture. So, I decided to do something about it. As a novice to core fitness, I started with crunches to strengthen my abs and began to see my posture improve. Anatomy and physiology classes have since taught me that the core is much more than abs, but it was a start. And I did begin to see a difference, not only in my posture, but also in my running.

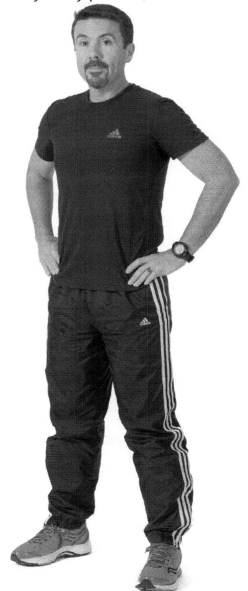

Runners entering their late 40s and early 50s can get discouraged when they start experiencing slower race times and waning endurance. Often they contribute it to age. While age is a factor, other factors may be greater contributors to these undesirable changes.

During our 20s and 30s, we're usually involved in many more athletic activities, such as swimming, tennis, volleyball, baseball, softball. Even if you weren't the jock type, you were probably playing with your kids, picking them up, toting them around on your hip and back, and doing yard work and other projects that involved the core and upper body. Without realizing it, these activities provided you with movements that helped keep your core and upper body conditioned.

As we get older, life gets in the way. We often have jobs that keep us slouched over a computer most of the day. There's less time for recreational sports, the kids are older, and there just doesn't seem to be enough time for fitness other than getting in a good run from time to time. As a result, the upper body becomes deconditioned. When your upper body and core lose that muscular endurance, fatigue creeps in a lot sooner, negatively affecting good running form. Poor running form is often the culprit in slowing down your pace.

When a runner experiencing this comes to me, I recommend full-body conditioning. This involves a series of circuit workouts composed of exercises designed to build full-body muscular endurance, with an extra focus on lateral movement of the lower body (to increase balance) and muscular endurance in the upper body and core. After a couple months of this, my client usually reports back with improved running form, pace, and endurance, particularly on longer runs.

One such client, Mike, makes annual visits to the prestigious Cooper Clinic in Dallas for an in-depth physical. After a year of working with Mike on full-body muscular endurance with a focus on the core, he received the following comment from Riva Rahl, MD, medical director of the clinic's Cooper Wellness lifestyle modification program (Dr. Rahl is also a 2:54 marathoner and the author of *Physical Activity and Health Guidelines* (Human Kinetics, 2010)):

"Michael, congratulations on having improved your stress test so significantly from last year. I think part of this may be due to the improved strength you have from the weight workouts and working out with a trainer [ED.: That's me!]. *I also think that the strength training has helped reduce your LDL to the best level it has been in several years. Great news! ... I think it is a good idea if you continue to do the weight workout with your trainer because this will also help maintain your core strength and will likely propel you to faster race times."*

As a runner for more than 25 years and having worked with hundreds of runners, I've seen again and again how full-body fitness—core, upper-body, and lower-body muscular endurance—can be the determining factor in setting that new PR or just regaining that lost running mojo.

The success of many of my clients is what spurred me on to write this book. Adding full-body fitness into your regular running routine can be easy and fun, and the benefits are many. It won't just help your running; it will also help to improve your overall quality of life.

The phrases "resistance training" or "lifting weights" can intimidate runners. Some worry about bulking up. Others worry it will take up more time that they already don't have. Still others are put off by the idea of joining a gym or purchasing expensive equipment.

This book will put those fears or hesitations to rest. You won't bulk up, the workouts take no more than 30 minutes, and with just a few pieces of inexpensive equipment, you can do the workouts at home.

Introduction

The workouts in *Full-Body Fitness for Runners* are designed to increase muscular endurance (muscles that will last for the long haul). Don't worry that you'll grow a 40-inch neck, bulging arms, or tree-trunk legs. That just won't happen. As for time, 30 minutes twice a week are all you need to make significant improvements in your overall fitness level. If you currently have a gym membership, that's great. Most gyms have the required equipment. Not a gym member? No worries. The workouts incorporate a few pieces of common exercise equipment: medicine ball, lightweight dumbbells, exercise bands and tubes, and a bench. You can easily find this gear at your local sporting goods or big-box discount store or through online outlets. A small initial investment will have you set up to do the workouts in the comfort of your own home.

There's no need to be intimidated by the workouts. Divided into three levels—novice, intermediate, and advanced—there's something for everyone. If you're new to fitness or unsure where to start, begin with the novice workouts. If you already have a moderate level of core and upper-body fitness, begin at the intermediate level. If you're a gym rat but don't know how to shoot specifically for muscular endurance, then try the advanced-level workouts.

The beauty of these workouts is that you can start at the novice level and work your way up to advanced. Once you've mastered all the levels, you can mix and match your favorite exercises from the various levels and create your own workouts. Just because an exercise is labeled "novice" doesn't mean it's not a great exercise to continue doing. Novice simply means that it's a good exercise for someone who's new to fitness.

Before beginning the exercises, I encourage you to read the book from beginning to end to learn more about the importance of full-body fitness for runners; the muscle groups involved in the upper body, core, and lower body; the importance of pre- and post-workout stretching; and proper fueling for your workouts.

You'll also find additional exercises that can be done with a partner, additional core exercises to throw into the mix, great running nutrition advice from Olympian Jeff Galloway, as well as some great pre- and post-workout fueling ideas, including some from such running notables as endurance athlete and best-selling author Dean Karnazes, ChiRunning founder Danny Dreyer, and international yoga expert and *Runner's World* columnist Sage Rountree, just to name a few.

Anatomy of a Runner

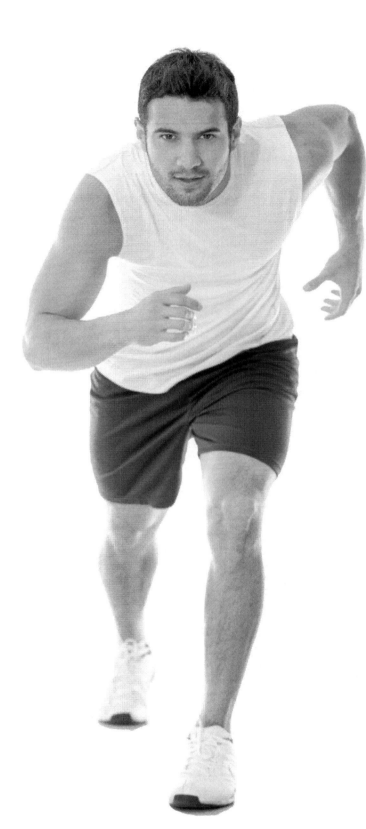

When it comes to running, legs are thought of as the big players. They are important, but you might be surprised to learn that it's more of a 50-50 relationship between upper body and lower body. The core might even play a more important role in running than the legs. A strong core aids in good posture and offers a solid base from which the rest of your body can properly do its job.

A weak core creates imbalance, putting extra strain on the posterior muscles and creating more work for the legs. This imbalance and extra work lead to quicker onset of muscle fatigue. Once the brain senses fatigue, it kicks in to "preservation mode," slowing the body as a means of protecting it.

Proper training, fueling, and hydration also play a role in preventing fatigue, but loss of good running form is often the culprit in endurance runners, particularly older runners. Muscular endurance in the chest, back, and arm muscles is also important. These muscles play a vital role in maintaining good running posture, especially during long endurance runs. A weak upper body can lead to a domino effect.

When the upper body (arms, chest, back) fatigues while running, it causes the runner to slouch and demands more from the core to maintain good running posture.

If the core is weak, it will soon fatigue as well. Before long the lower body is doing double duty to pick up the slack. Ever see a runner near the end of a marathon bent over at the waist, struggling to make it to the finish? Chances are he's in the final stage of this domino effect.

Core refers to a lot more than just beach-body six-pack abs. To optimize core strength, a six-pack shouldn't be the goal. Instead, strive for a solid core—360 degrees. If you get a "pack" in the process, that's just a bonus. (I'm still waiting for mine.) Instead of core, think torso: front, sides, and back.

Don't neglect the legs, however; quad dominance often results in endurance runners, particularly those who overstride. While the quads will always be stronger than hamstrings, too much of an imbalance can set up a runner for injury. Overstriding (where the foot lands well ahead of the torso) causes a runner to activate the quads to pull the body forward. Over time this constant pulling motion and overdevelopment of the quads can lead to an imbalance between the front and back of the upper leg.

Running should be more of a push than a pull-then-push. Striving for a midfoot (that is, flat-footed) landing under your center of mass will help decrease the chance of overdeveloping your quads. As a bonus, it increases your running efficiency. Less quad activation means less caloric burn. Less caloric burn means more fuel for the long haul. It also helps delay the onset of fatigue.

Meet Your Muscles

Upper Body

Pectoralis major ("pecs"): Fanning out across the chest from sternum to upper arm, this muscle flexes, internally rotates, and brings the arm toward the body.

Deltoids ("delts"): Divided into three sections—rear, middle, and front—this group of shoulder muscles raises the arm (anterior delt), abducts or lifts the arm away from the body (middle delt), and extends or moves the shoulder backward (rear delt).

Triceps: Running along the back of the upper arm, this muscle works to extend the arm at the elbow. Without the triceps, you wouldn't be able to straighten your arm.

Biceps: Running along the front of the upper and lower arm, this muscle group flexes the arm at the elbow so you can bend your arm and rotate the lower arm.

Trapezius ("traps"): Found along the upper back, the traps raise, rotate, and retract the scapula, making it possible to lift, abduct, and retract the shoulders.

Core

Latissimus dorsi ("lats"): Running from the bottom half of the spine and upper posterior iliac crest (back of the pelvis bone) to the upper arm, this large fan-shaped muscle pulls the upper arm down and back and helps pull the arm toward the body.

Rectus abdominis ("abs"): Running from the lower rib cage and sternum, down the torso to the pubic bone, this muscle helps flex the trunk (bend it forward).

External obliques: Extending from the crest of the ilium to the pectorals, these outer abdominal muscles help rotate the trunk and pull the chest downward.

Internal obliques: Beneath the external obliques and running in the opposite direction, these muscles help flex and rotate the torso. The right internal oblique works with the left external oblique when flexing and rotating the torso.

Erector spinae: Running along the spine from your neck to your lower back, this group of muscles stabilizes the spine and helps to extend the spine, allowing it to arch backward.

Multifidus: A small but powerful muscle found deep beneath the erector spinae in the lower back that supports the spine.

Transverse abdominis: Located deep below the internal obliques, this muscle runs laterally across the abdomen and works like a natural "weight belt" to provide pelvic stability.

Lower Body

Hip flexors: Found in front of the pelvis and upper thigh, this group of muscles flexes the femur.

Gluteus maximus: Found at the back of the hip, this muscle helps extend and laterally rotate the hip.

Hip adductors: Running along the inner thigh, this group of muscles pulls the leg inward toward the body.

Hip abductors: These muscles along the hip pull the leg away from the body.

Hamstrings: Running along the back of the upper leg, this group of three muscles works together to flex the knee and extend the hip.

Quadriceps ("quads"): Running down the front of the thigh and merging together at the kneecap, this group of four muscles works to extend the knee.

Tibialis anterior: Running along the outer portion of the shin, this muscle works to raise the foot toward the upper leg.

Calves: Running along the back of the lower leg, this group of two muscles allows for plantar flexion (rising up on your toes).

The Runner's Front

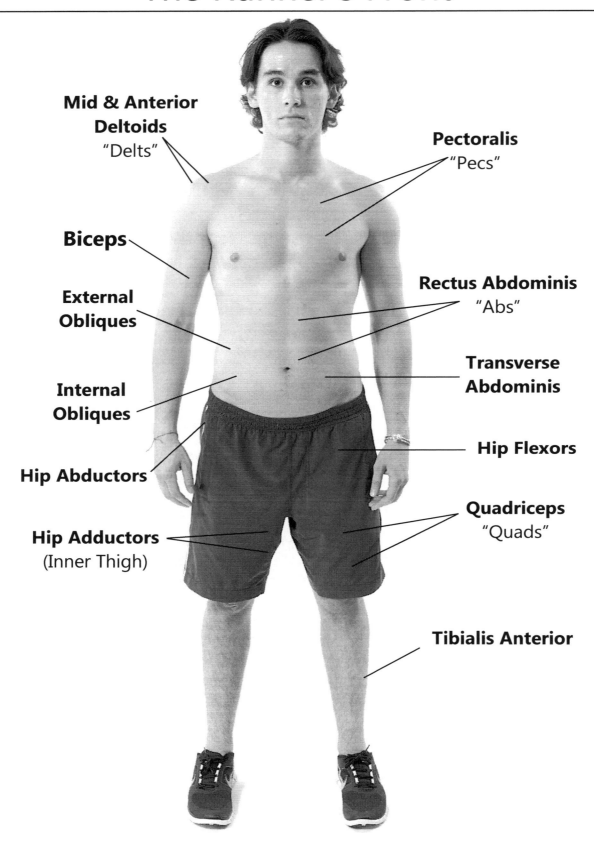

Mid & Anterior Deltoids
"Delts"

Pectoralis
"Pecs"

Biceps

Rectus Abdominis
"Abs"

External Obliques

Internal Obliques

Transverse Abdominis

Hip Abductors

Hip Flexors

Hip Adductors
(Inner Thigh)

Quadriceps
"Quads"

Tibialis Anterior

The Runner's Back

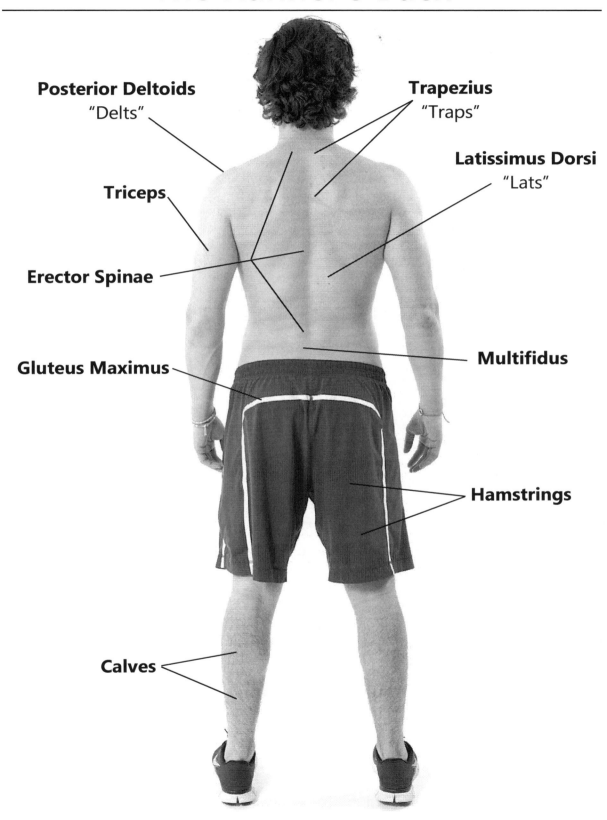

Posterior Deltoids
"Delts"

Trapezius
"Traps"

Triceps

Latissimus Dorsi
"Lats"

Erector Spinae

Gluteus Maximus

Multifidus

Hamstrings

Calves

Five Steps to Getting Started

1. Get a checkup. Before beginning these workouts, meet with your physician and discuss what you're planning to do. A clean bill of health will give you peace of mind before starting a new fitness regimen.

2. Schedule it. Getting started is the hardest part of any new routine. Success comes with consistency. Consistency comes with treating the new activity like anything else in your workday. Schedule it. If you plan to run or work out during your lunch hour, add it to your calendar as a meeting. That way your colleagues will see that you're busy, and you'll be less likely to get pulled into other meetings. At home, before or after work, pick times when you're less likely to be disturbed. (See pages 107–109 for tips on how to fit the workouts into your busy schedule.)

3. Share your goal. The most important thing to do before getting started is to let your coworkers, friends, and family know your plans. Making them aware and getting their support can have a huge positive effect on your success. Not only will their support be encouraging, but it will also boost your level of accountability.

4. Be prepared. Once you've created your workout schedule and have everyone on board, make sure you have the proper workout attire and equipment. Adopt the "no excuses" approach to working out. If you're working out at the office or in a gym, pack a backup bag to keep at your desk or in the trunk of your car. Don't keep your best workout clothes or shoes in this bag, but do pack gear that you don't mind being seen in while working out. If you forget your workout clothes or running shoes, you'll have no excuse for skipping your workout.

5. Take inventory. Take a look at the equipment you currently have, and make a list of the items you need to perform your workouts. In the next section, you'll find descriptions of all the equipment needed for the workouts in this book. If you plan to work out at the gym, bring this book and ask the manager if the gym has everything you'll need. If you plan to work out at home, you can purchase the items at most sporting goods or big-box department stores, and be sure to check websites like Amazon.com for great deals.

Medicine Ball

Medicine balls are weighted balls about the size of a basketball or smaller. Some contain air and bounce somewhat like a basketball. Others are soft and filled with sand. Medicine balls come in weights ranging from two to 20 or more pounds. For the exercises in this book, you'll need a six- to 10-pound ball. If you're new to fitness, a six-pound ball is a good start.

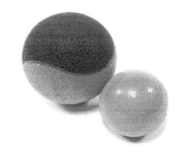

Stability Ball

Sometimes called a Swiss ball, balance ball, physio ball, or exercise ball, a stability ball is great for adding a balance element to most any exercise that's typically performed on a weight bench.

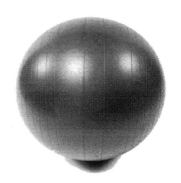

Resistance Bands and Tubes

Resistance bands are typically strips of stretchy elastic material that can be used as a strip or tied together in a loop to add resistance to exercise movements. Resistance tubes are usually sturdier than bands and have handles. Most resistance bands and tubes come in light, medium, and heavy resistance.

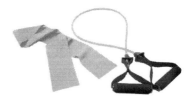

Dumbbells

For the exercises in this book, light dumbbells ranging from five to 15 pounds will suffice.

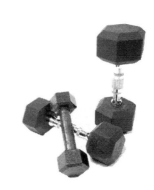

Exercise Mat

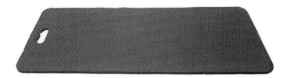

Exercise mats come in many different lengths and thicknesses. Yoga mats tend to be long and thin. Exercise mats tend to be shorter and slightly thicker. Yoga mats can be folded over for extra thickness, if needed. An exercise mat provides protection when doing floor exercises. If working out at home, a padded carpeted area will also work.

Exercise Bench

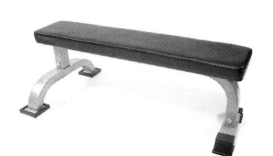

An exercise bench is optional. A sturdy chair, low table, or even the floor can be a good alternative. If you use a table or chair, be sure it's stable and sturdy enough to hold your body weight. A stability ball or exercise step can also be used in place of an exercise bench.

Exercise Step

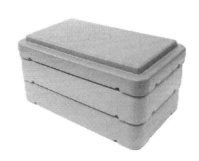

Exercise steps are optional equipment. Stairs in your home are a good alternative. The benefit of exercise steps, however, is that they are often adjustable and can be raised or lowered to increase or decrease difficulty.

Balance Disk

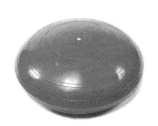

Balance disks are optional equipment. They are available in various shapes and sizes. Some are filled with air while others are hard and flat. Balance disks are great for turning any exercise into a full-body exercise. Standing on a balance disk while exercising recruits core and leg-stabilizer muscles.

Acclimation

You've seen it many times with family, friends, and colleagues, and you may have experienced it yourself: You enter a new fitness program with excitement and expectations of quick results, but a day or two after that first workout, you're sore and tired. You stay sore and tired for the next week. Week two isn't much better. You get discouraged. You're thinking, "I feel worse than before I started. What's the point?" This is the "make or break" point for most of us.

What most people don't know is that what they're feeling is normal. No matter your fitness level, whether you're just off the couch or an Olympic athlete, when you add new intensities to your current fitness level, your body feels it and experiences a period of acclimation. This acclimation period is called the **gain threshold**.

Basically, your body needs time to acclimate to the new demands you're putting on it. Your mind and body are going through a learning curve. Your mind is learning how to persevere. Your body is learning how to work hard and rebuild.

The Gain Threshold

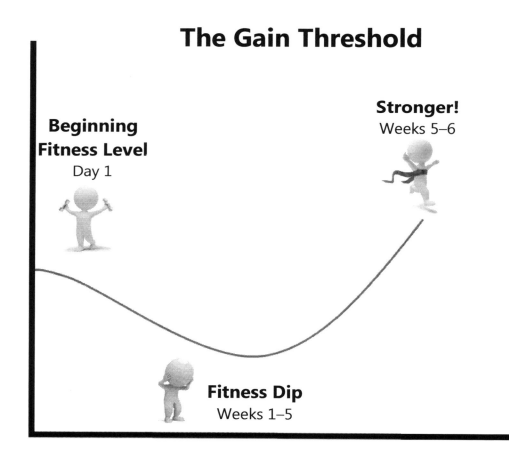

Beginning Fitness Level
Day 1

Stronger!
Weeks 5–6

Fitness Dip
Weeks 1–5

This acclimation period may take anywhere from four to six weeks before you begin to feel stronger than when you started your fitness quest. A person with a higher fitness level may take less time to pull out of the gain threshold than a less fit individual, but both will feel the drain of the new demands on the body.

Seasoned endurance runners are often surprised how sore they are after adding weekly full-body fitness workouts to their normal routine. Keep in mind that your body is going to react to any new intensities you put on it. So while your body might be conditioned to run 10 miles, it might not be conditioned to the new core exercises you're putting it through.

The good news is that this gain threshold or "fitness dip" is short term. It will get better. If you hang tough, fuel properly, keep the new workouts going, and get ample rest, you will pull out of this dip and begin feeling stronger than when you started.

Setting realistic expectations is key when beginning any new fitness or running program. If you enter your new fitness regimen expecting some initial discomfort, it won't be as much of a shock that day or two after your first couple of workouts when you find it hard to crawl into or out of bed.

The following tips will help ease you through the acclimation phase.

Work out with a buddy. Seeing someone else experiencing the same initial aches and pains will reassure you that it's "not just you." Encouraging each other can be extremely motivating during those first few weeks.

Fuel your workouts. Giving your body enough fuel to sustain activity will greatly improve the quality of your workouts. Refueling within 30 minutes after every workout provides the nutrients your body needs to begin rebuilding quickly, which in turn helps to ease post-workout discomfort. Be sure to keep the caloric intake of your pre- and post-workout fueling appropriate. (See pages 129–131 for healthy snack ideas.)

Set realistic goals. A beach-body six-pack in a month isn't realistic. Give yourself that month to work on becoming consistent with your new fitness routine and acclimating to the new demands you're putting on your body. Don't get discouraged if the fruits of your labor are not immediately apparent.

Learn to celebrate the small gains. Celebrate the first day you wake up without soreness, or when you increase your reps for an exercise, or when you realize your balance has improved for an exercise that's been difficult. Small improvements lead to huge gains over time.

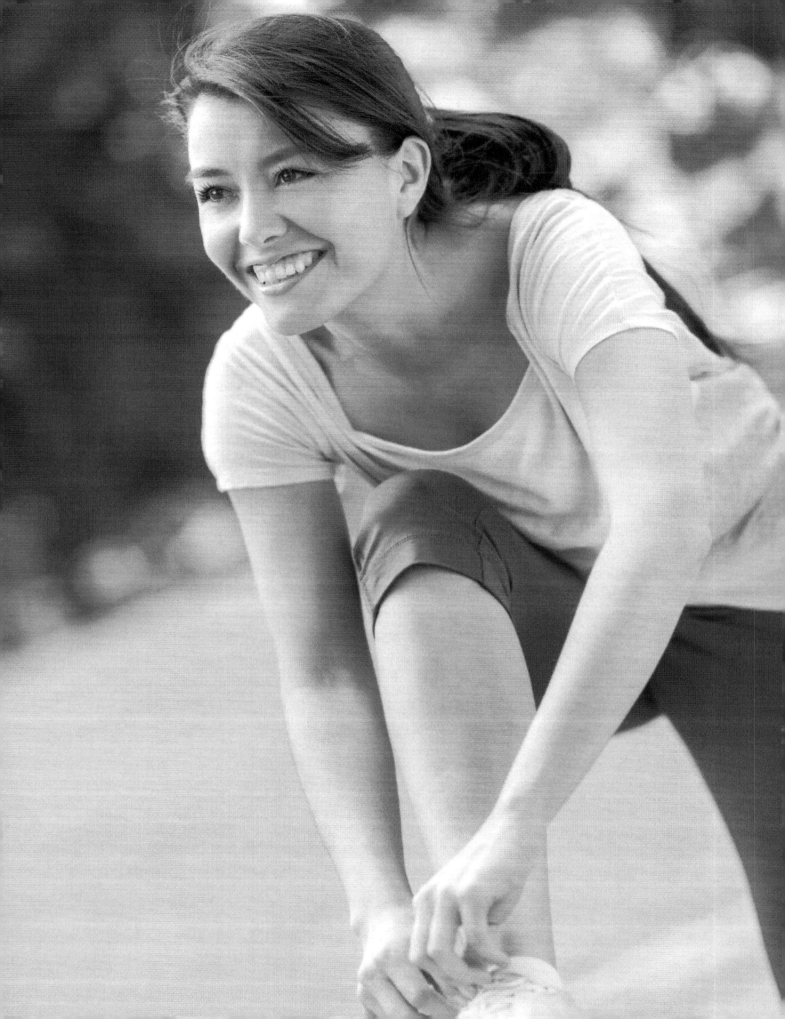

10 Tips for New Runners

1. Purchase running shoes. This seems like a no-brainer, but starting to run with the right pair of shoes can help head off possible injury. The sneakers you've been knocking around in for the past two years are great for just that—knocking around in. The best thing to do is visit your local, independently owned running store and have them fit you for running shoes. Tell them you're a new runner and that you're not sure what you need, and ask them to analyze your gait and determine the best shoe for you.

2. Go technical. Invest in some technical-fabric running shorts, tops, and socks. Technical fabrics are made of materials that are natural (bamboo, merino wool), synthetic (polyester, nylon, Lycra), or a combination of both. Avoid 100 percent cotton, which tends to retain moisture, causing chafing, irritation, and even blisters. Technical fabrics allow moisture to rise to the surface, where it can evaporate.

3. Find a group. Joining a running group or running with a buddy dramatically increases motivation, inspiration, accountability, and commitment. Everyone experiences days when they don't want to run, but having buddies counting on you can make all the difference in whether you hit the snooze button or get out of bed and join them. Check with your local running store. Many host beginning running groups or know coaches in the area who work with beginning runners.

4. Get a plan. Just stepping out the door and running does not work for many of us, especially if you've been sedentary or away from exercise for a while. Following a beginning running plan, such as a run/walk plan, will provide structure and guidance and help take the guesswork out of what to do and how to do it.

5. Acclimate. Whenever you begin new exercise, your fitness level will actually dip a little while you acclimate to the new demands you're putting on your body. This is when most new runners give up. Anticipating that "fitness dip" can lessen the shock during those first couple weeks of running. Hang in there, and before you know it you'll pull out of that dip and begin to feel stronger than before you started. (See pages 24–25 for more information on acclimation.)

6. Fuel up. Fueling your new activity is very important. Timing is key. A good rule of thumb is to eat about 200 to 400 calories of mostly complex carbs and a little protein about 90 minutes prior to your run. This will give your body time to digest the food and acquire the necessary energy for your activity. (See pages 112–113 and 129-131 for more tips on pre- and post-run fueling.)

7. Drink up. Being well hydrated is just as important as being well fueled. Drink about 20 ounces of water about two hours prior to running. This will give it time to pass through your system and be voided before your run.

8. Warm up. Before you head out on your run, be sure to warm up your muscles. A five-minute walk is a great warm-up. This will help decrease the chance of muscle tightness during your run. Save the traditional stretch-and-hold stretches for after your run.

9. Get in tune with your body. Listen to your body. If you're feeling something other than regular workout-related muscle soreness, don't run. Running through pain is never a good idea. If you're experiencing pain along the shin, hip, iliotibial (IT) band, or any area of the body that's beyond normal muscle soreness, ice it, elevate it, take your usual choice of anti-inflammatory medication, and rest. When you no longer feel any pain, ease back into your running. Use the following 10-point pain scale to help evaluate any pain you're experiencing:

- **Mild pain (rating 1–3):** The type of pain you feel when you start to exercise, but it usually goes away as you start to warm up and continue running. The pain may be inconsistent and move around the body, or you may feel it bilaterally, which means you feel it in the same joints in both limbs, such as in both knees. Mild pain or discomfort is common for new runners and considered safe to run through. After your run, place ice on any sore areas. A bag of frozen peas works really well.

- **Moderate pain (rating 4–6):** Pain at this level is more than mild pain, but it's not enough to cause a limp or alter your stride. Typically, a few days of rest, low-impact cross-training, and icing as needed will help. If it doesn't, go see the doc.

- **Severe pain (rating 7–10):** Pain at this level requires immediate medical attention. This kind of pain you feel before, during, and after the run. It usually starts at the beginning of a run and increases until your stride is altered or you stop. Don't let it get that far.

10. Rest. Rest is just as important as your workout. It allows your body time to rebuild and recover. When you run or exercise, you actually create micro-tears in the muscle tissue, and your body rushes in to repair the tissue. This is the normal muscle-building process that makes you stronger. If you don't take the proper rest, however, your body might not have time to fully repair before your next run, causing you to feel sore, tired, and sluggish. When you first start a running program, it's a good idea to include at least one day of rest between every run.

Stretching

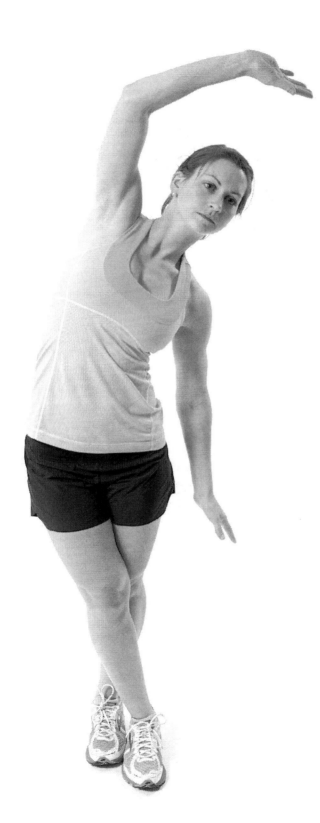

Stretching is very important, but runners often neglect it. Before working out or running, active stretching is best. Active or dynamic stretching is basically moving the body in the manner in which it's getting ready to be used. So, for running, an easy walk or slow jog of five to 10 minutes before the actual run is usually enough. The same goes for working out: Hop on the treadmill or elliptical machine for five to 10 minutes or take a walk around the block before your workout.

After your warm-up walk/run, if you still feel tight in a particular area, such as the calves or quads, feel free to do some traditional static stretches (stretch-and-hold stretches); however, these are best saved for after your workout or run.

If you're planning to do an intense speed workout like hill repeats or intervals, follow up the initial easy walk/run with some butt kicks, high knee raises, walking lunges, skipping, and/or side shuffles to further warm up and stretch your muscles.

Active Stretch

(Before a Workout or Run)

Lunge with Reverse Fly

Stand with a tall spine. Step forward with your right leg while pulling your arms down and back (see figure A). Be sure to keep a neutral spine. Do not bend forward at the waist. Return to a standing position. Repeat with the left leg.

Repeat again, but this time pull your arms back and out to the sides of your body, making the letter T (see figure B).

Repeat a third time with both legs while raising your arms above your head, making the letter Y (see figure C).

Continue lunging, alternating legs, while cycling through the three arm positions for 30 seconds.

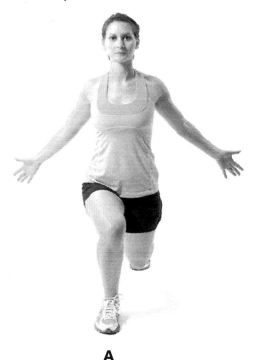

A

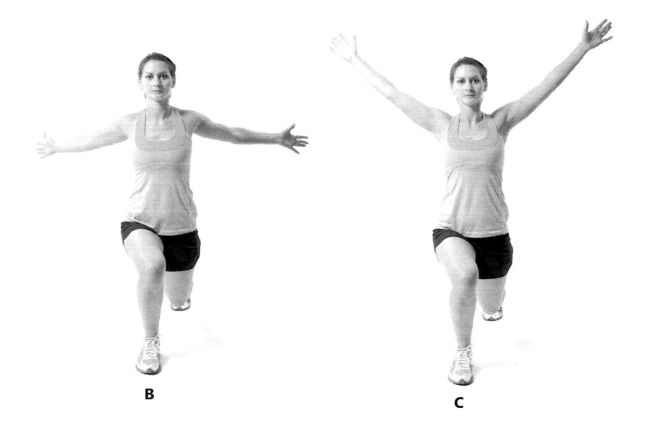

B

C

Lower-Body Static Stretches
(After a Workout or Run)

Adductors (Inner Thigh) Stretch

Sit on your bottom with the soles of your feet touching. Grab your lower legs with your hands while placing your elbows on your knees. Allow the weight of your elbows to gently press down on the insides of your knees. As you apply this gentle pressure, you'll feel a stretch along the inner thigh. This is also good for stretching the groin muscles and hips. Hold for about 30 seconds.

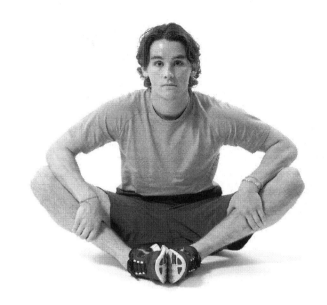

Hamstring Stretch

This stretch is great not only for the hamstrings, but also the glutes and piriformis. To perform the stretch, lie on your back. Raise both legs in the air. Then cross the left leg over the right knee. Reach around the right leg as shown and pull it gently toward your chest. You'll feel a stretch along the hamstrings and glutes of the left leg. Hold for about 30 seconds, then repeat with the other leg.

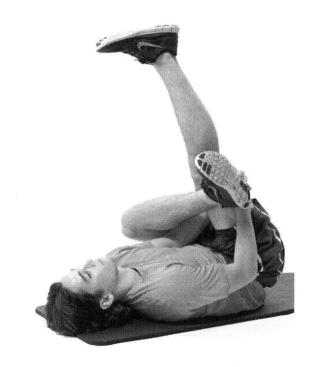

The following two stretches are great for stretching the hip muscle (glute medius). Tight hip muscles can pull on the iliotibial (IT) band, causing tightness down the outer part of the thigh. Tight IT bands are often the cause of runner's knee.

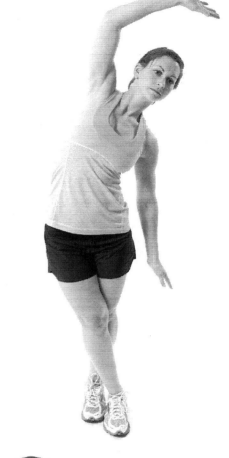

Hip Stretch #1

Stand tall. Cross the right leg over the left. Raise your right arm above your torso and slowly bend your body toward the left. As you bend, gently lift the right shoulder until you feel a stretch in the right hip. Hold for 30 seconds. Repeat with the other side.

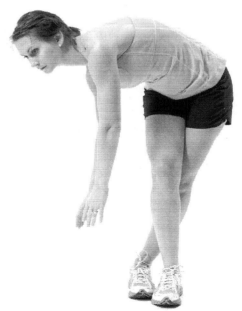

Hip Stretch #2

Stand tall. Cross the left leg behind the right. While bending at the waist, slowly lower both hands toward your right foot. As you reach for your right foot, raise your left shoulder until you feel a stretch in the left hip. Hold for 30 seconds. Repeat with the other side.

Quad Stretch

Lie face down on a mat. Reach back with your right hand and grab your right foot as shown. Gently pull your foot toward your buttocks. If you're unable to reach your foot, loop a towel or belt around your foot. Hold for 30 seconds. Repeat with the other side.

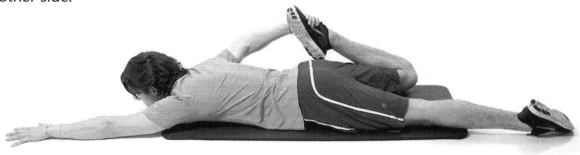

For an even better stretch, try grabbing both feet.

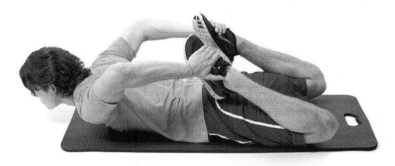

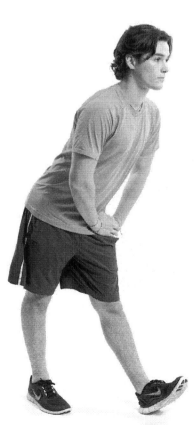

Calf Stretch

Place the right foot perpendicular to your body. Extend your left leg out in front of you with your left heel on the floor and your left knee locked. Put your hands in the fold of your left leg as shown. Gently bend forward while pulling the toes of your left foot toward you. Hold for 30 seconds. Repeat with the other side. To get an even better calf stretch, rotate the foot from side to side while lifting the toes.

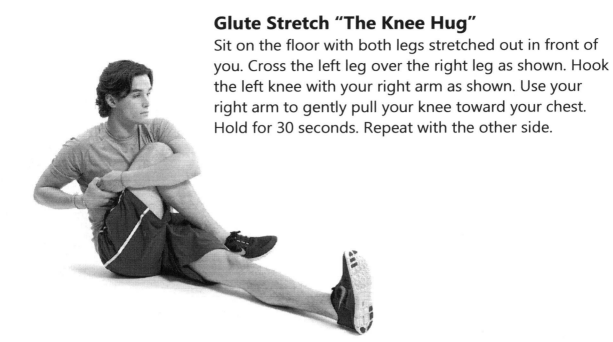

Glute Stretch "The Knee Hug"

Sit on the floor with both legs stretched out in front of you. Cross the left leg over the right leg as shown. Hook the left knee with your right arm as shown. Use your right arm to gently pull your knee toward your chest. Hold for 30 seconds. Repeat with the other side.

Tibialis Anterior Stretch

Sit on the floor with both legs stretched out in front of you. Grab your right foot and gently pull it toward your chest as shown so that the bottom of your right foot is facing you. This will stretch the tibialis anterior muscle, which runs along the outer portion of the shin in your lower leg.

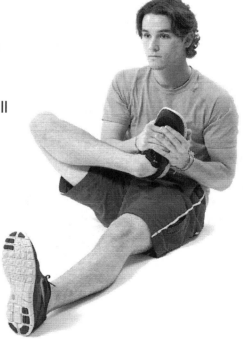

Upper-Body Static Stretches

(After a Workout or Run)

Shoulder and Upper-Back Stretch

Stand with a tall spine. Place your right arm across your chest. Use your left hand to pull your right arm closer to your chest. You should feel a stretch in your right shoulder and upper back. Hold for 30 seconds. Repeat with your left arm across your chest.

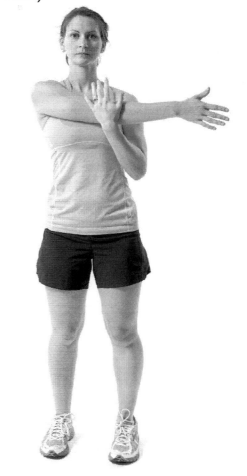

Latissimus Dorsi Stretch

Kneel in front of a set of stacked exercise steps (a weight bench or stability ball will also work). There should be about three feet between the steps and your knees. Lean forward, bending at the waist, and place both hands on the steps. While keeping your hands positioned on the steps, slowly lower your torso so that your head dips below your arms. You should feel the stretch in the lats along both sides and the middle of your back. To focus on just one side of the lats, place just one hand on the steps.

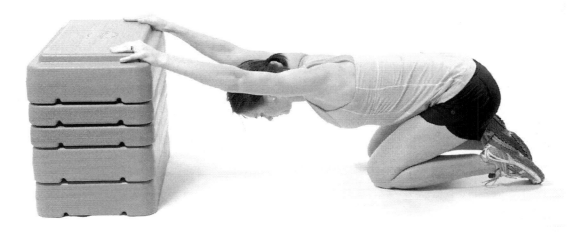

Biceps Stretch

Extend your right arm in front of your torso with the palm facing up. Grab your right hand with your left hand and gently pull the right hand back as shown. Hold for 30 seconds. Repeat with the other side. This stretch is subtler than other stretches, but it's effective in loosening the biceps muscles.

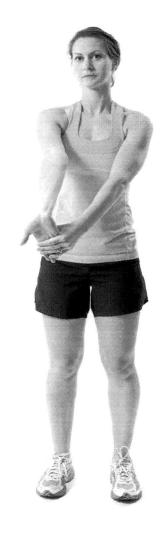

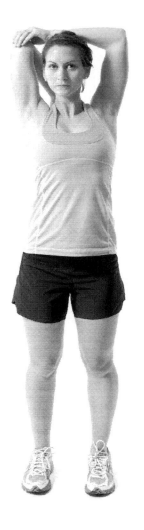

Triceps Stretch

Stand with a tall spine. Reach your left hand over your head and pull your right elbow back as shown. You'll feel a stretch in the back of the upper right arm. Hold for 30 seconds. Repeat with the other side.

Abdominal and Oblique Stretch

Lay supine over a stability ball with your arms fully extended behind your head. Reach back as far as you can until you feel a nice stretch along the abdominal muscles. Hold for 30 seconds. To stretch the obliques and the sides of your abdomen, reach toward one side and hold for 30 seconds. Then reach for the opposite side and hold for 30 seconds.

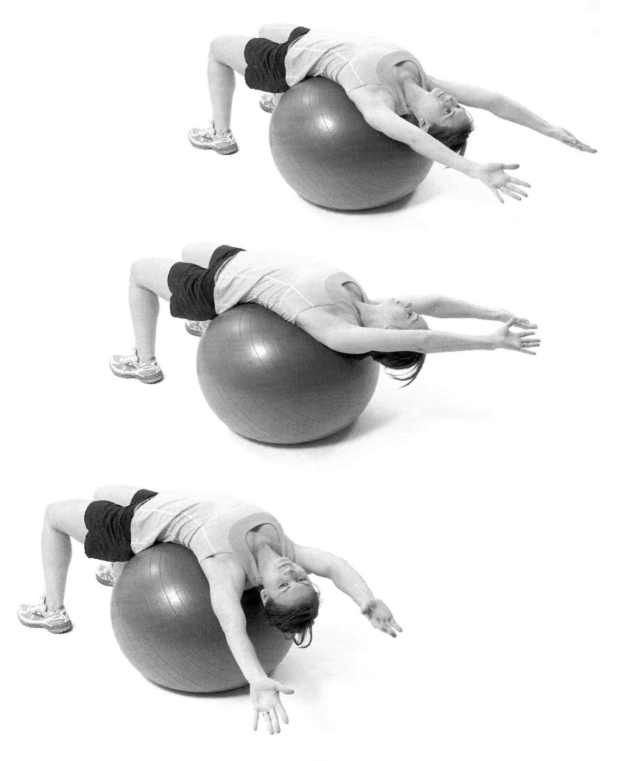

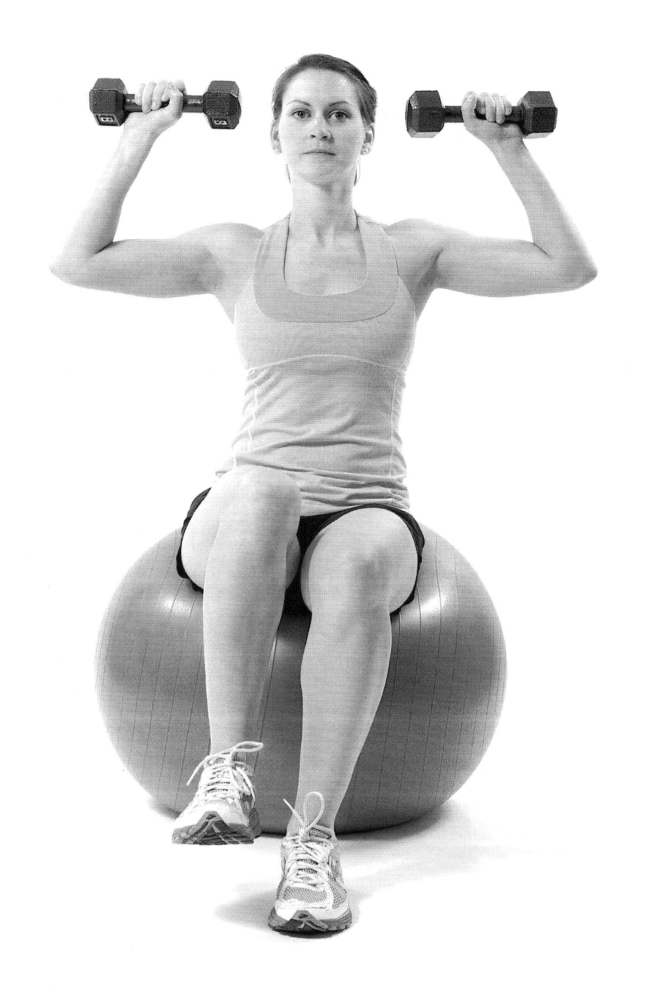

How to Complete the Workouts

One misconception about fitness is that it takes a lot of time. When it comes to fitness, quality trumps quantity. Consistency is key. A focused 30-minute workout circuit performed two to three times a week is sufficient for most runners to begin seeing substantial improvements in their running. No worries about being stuck in a gym for hours.

Traditional workouts designed to add bulk usually consist of performing an exercise with heavier weights for eight to 10 reps (one set), then resting for several minutes before repeating two more sets. That's why most of us think working out takes so long. Imagine doing that for 12 exercises. You *would* be in the gym for hours. Unless your goal is bodybuilding, there's no need to spend that much time with each exercise.

A runner's goal is to create muscular endurance (lasting muscles), not hypertrophy (adding bulk). The following workouts have you using body weight and lighter weights with higher repetitions. The circuit design eliminates much of the rest associated with more traditional workouts. With each circuit, you move from one exercise to the next without a rest break. Rest comes at the end of the circuit before you begin a second round of the exercises. Moving from one exercise to the next without rest adds an aerobic component to the workouts, which helps increase stamina and cardio strength.

The workouts are divided into lower-body/core and upper-body/core circuits. If you're new to circuit training, start with two workouts a week—one upper-body/core workout and one lower-body/core workout. Include at least one day of rest between workouts.

There are three workout levels: novice, intermediate, and advanced. As you acclimate and become stronger, you can increase the intensity by moving to the next level of workouts. You can also increase the intensity within your workout level by slightly increasing the weight used in the exercise, increasing the repetitions, or adding a third round of the circuit.

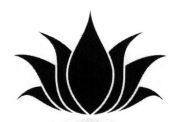

Lower Body/Core Workouts

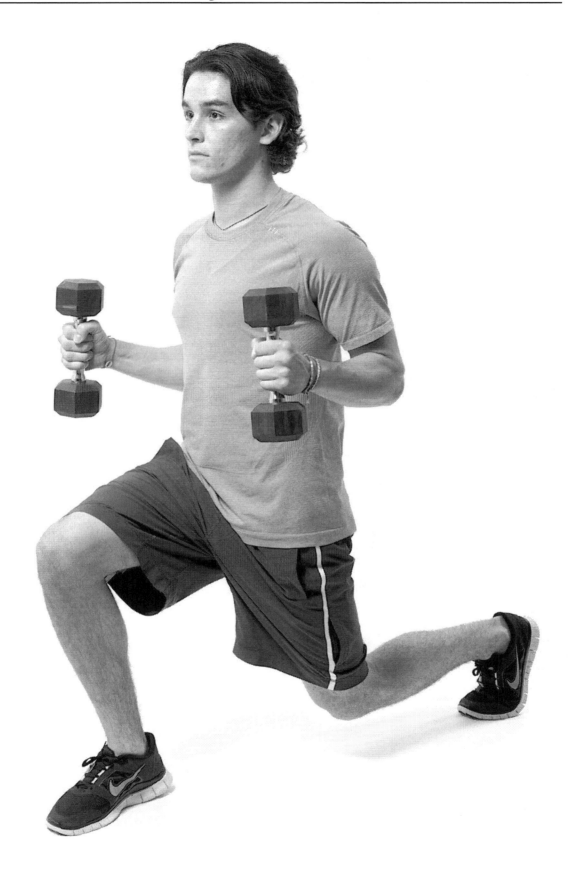

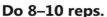

1. Medicine Ball Side-Middle-Side Crunch
Target Muscles: Rectus Abdominis, Internal and External Obliques

Lie flat on the floor with your legs spread in a wide V. Position a medicine ball above your right shoulder. Grab the ball with both hands. Keeping your arms fully extended, lift your arms and torso, moving the ball forward until it touches the floor between your legs. Lift the ball back over your left shoulder as you slowly lower your torso back to the floor. This is one rep.
Do 8–10 reps.

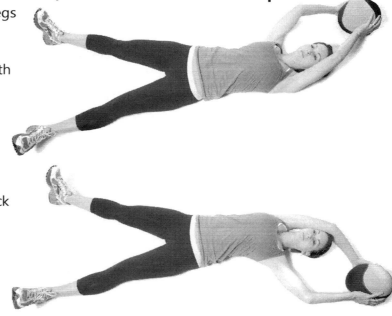

2. Stability Ball Wall Squat
Target Muscles: Quads, Gluteus Maximus

Grasp a dumbbell in each hand. Then position a stability ball between the small of your back and a wall. Lean against the ball. Place your feet ahead of your torso a little more than shoulder width apart. While holding the dumbbells by your sides, slowly bend your knees, lowering your body until your upper legs are parallel to the floor. Return to standing. This is one rep.
Do 8–10 reps.

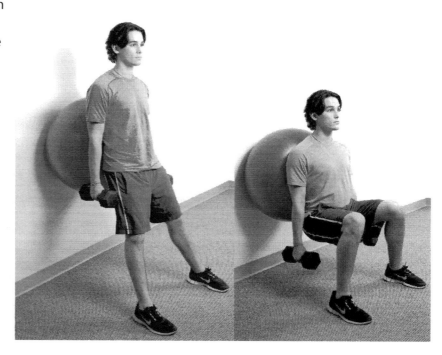

3. Anchored Reverse Crunch
Target Muscles: Rectus Abdominis

Place a heavy dumbbell on the floor. Lie on the floor with the dumbbell positioned above your head. Use the dumbbell as an anchor by reaching behind your head and grasping the dumbbell with both hands. Keeping your feet together, lift them as you bend your knees to 90 degrees. Engage the core and pull your knees toward your chest. Continue until your bottom is a few inches off the floor. Slowly return your bottom to the floor. That's one rep.

Do 8–10 reps.

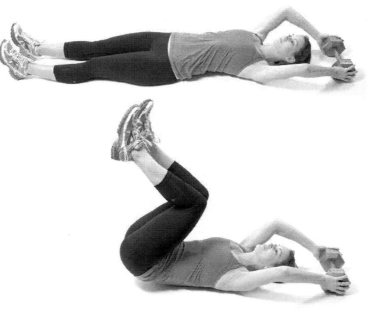

4. Elevated Hamstring Leg Lift
Target Muscles: Hamstrings, Gluteus Maximus

Lie on a mat with both feet resting on the edge of a bench or exercise step. Raise your right leg while keeping the left foot on the step. Use the left leg to raise your body off the mat until your body is a straight line from your left knee to your shoulder, then lower your body until it almost touches the floor. That's one rep.

Do 8–10 reps.

Repeat the process with the right foot on the step and the left leg in the air.

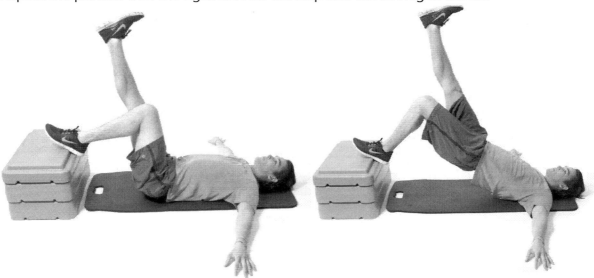

5. Superman
Target Muscles: Erector Spinae, Gluteus Maximus

Lie face down on a mat with both arms fully extended above your head and resting on the floor. Simultaneously lift both arms and both legs. Hold this position for a count of five, then lower your arms and legs back to the floor. That's one rep.

Do 8–10 reps.

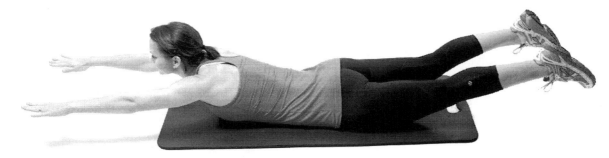

6. Dumbbell Farmer's Walk
Target Muscle: Calves

Hold a dumbbell at each side. Keeping the knees locked, lift your heels and walk around on your toes for 30 to 60 seconds.

Note: This is also very effective without weights.

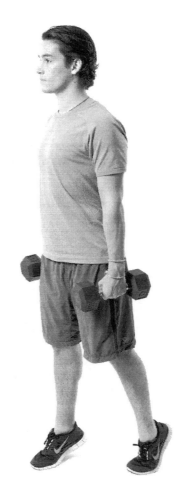

Lower Body/Core Workout <u>**NOVICE**</u>

7. Mountain Climber
Target Muscles: Full Body

Begin in a push-up position with each hand gripping a dumbbell and your legs in a staggered stance with the right foot on the floor underneath your chest and your left leg extended behind your torso with only your toes on the floor. To begin the exercise, quickly lift both feet and switch positions, bringing the left foot forward up toward the chest and moving the right foot back and fully extending the right leg. Continue alternating the feet in this back-and-forth motion for 30 seconds.

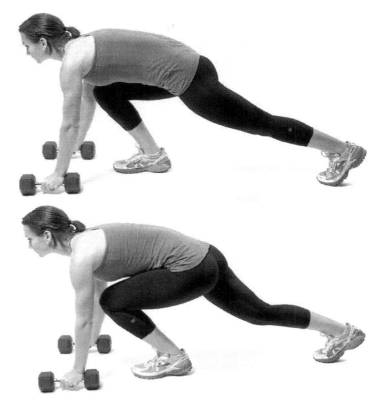

8. Resistance Band Clamshell
Target Muscles: Gluteus Medius

Tie an exercise band around both legs and position it just above your knees. Lie on your side and stack your feet. Bend both legs at the knee. Keeping the feet stacked, raise the top leg as far as you can, then lower it. That's one rep.

Do 8–10 reps.

Flip over and repeat the process with the other leg.

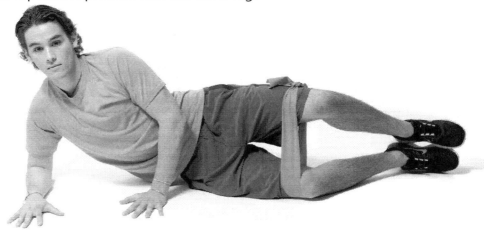

9. Stability Ball–Medicine Ball Crunch

Target Muscles: Rectus Abdominis

Sit on a stability ball holding a medicine ball with both hands at chest level. Roll out so that the small of your back is resting on the stability ball. Engage the core and crunch forward to a sitting position. Be sure to raise the torso without rocking back on your heels. Only your upper body should move, not your legs. Slowly return to the starting position. That's one rep.

Do 8–10 reps.

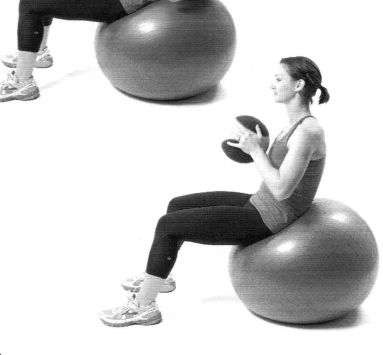

10. Slider Hip Adduction

Target Muscles: Adductors

Rest each knee on a Gliding Disc*. Slowly slide your knees about a foot apart, then slowly slide both knees back to the starting position. That's one rep.

Do 8–10 reps.

Paper plates or furniture movers also work well on hard and carpeted surfaces.

*You can purchase Gliding Discs at www.power-systems.com.

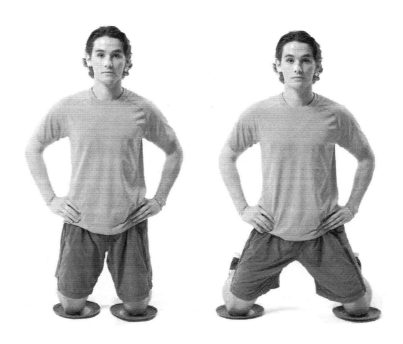

Lower Body/Core Workout **NOVICE**

11. Knee Tiger Plank

Target Muscles: Traps, Lats, Erector Spinae, Multifidus, Hip Extensors, Glutes

Position yourself on the floor in "all fours" (on hands and knees). Make sure your hands are under your shoulders and your knees are under your hips. Your back should be a straight plank. Simultaneously raise your left arm and extend your right leg. Hold for a count of two, then return your arm and leg to the starting position and repeat with the right arm and left leg. Continue alternating raising and extending the opposite arm and leg for 30 seconds.

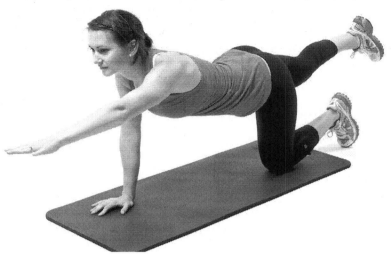

12. Dumbbell Jump Squat

Target Muscles: Hamstrings, Glutes, Quads

Holding a light dumbbell at each side, lower your body into a squat position. Be sure your knees are in line with or behind your toes. Also make sure that you're looking forward, not down, and that you have a neutral spine. You should not be bent over at the waist. From this squat position, explosively jump straight up. That's one rep. Upon landing, go directly into the squat position and repeat.

Do 8–10 reps.

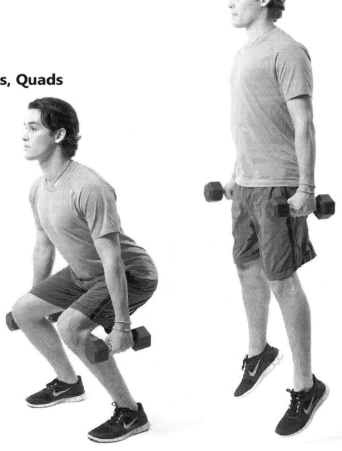

1. Bicycle Crunch

Target Muscles: Internal and External Obliques

Lie on your back, knees bent and hands beside your ears. Gently raise your shoulders off the floor, creating an isometric hold with your abdomen. Next, bring your right elbow and left knee toward each other as you fully extend the right leg. Repeat with the left elbow and right leg while extending the left leg. That's one rep.

Do 10–12 reps.

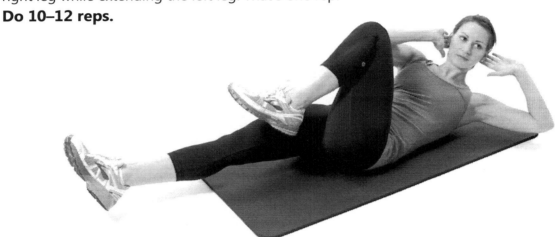

2. Offset Dumbbell Lunge

Target Muscles: Quads, Core

With a bent arm and neutral grip, hold a dumbbell by your right shoulder. Stand tall with your feet about shoulder-width apart. Engage your core as you step forward with your right leg. When your foot lands, slowly drop your hips until your right thigh is parallel with the floor. Your left calf should also be parallel with the floor. Check that your right knee is in line with the end of your toes (or just behind them). This is one rep.

Do 10–12 reps.

Switch the dumbbell to your left hand and repeat with the left foot stepping forward.

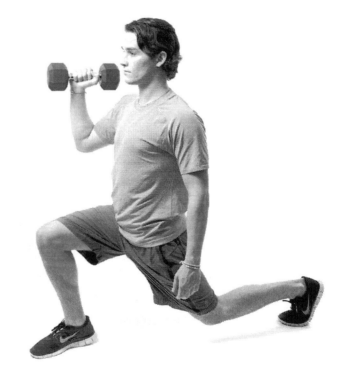

Lower Body/Core Workout

3. Cross-Leg Reverse Crunch

Target Muscles: Rectus Abdominis

Lie on the floor with both legs raised and your arms stretched out beside your torso. Cross your left leg over the right leg. Engage the core and lift your bottom off the floor. Slowly lower your bottom to the floor. This is one rep.

Do 10–12 reps.

Repeat with your right leg crossed and left leg extended.

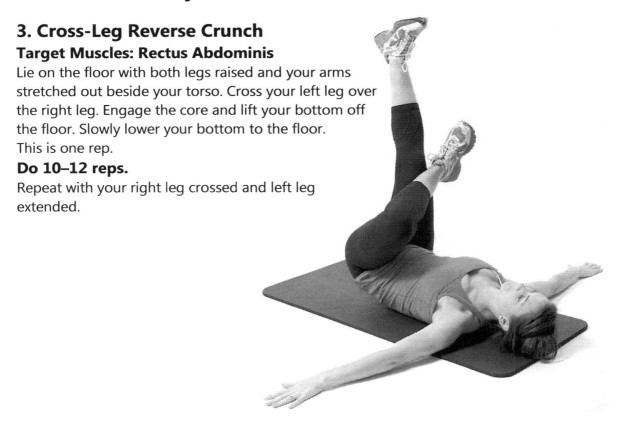

4. Stability Ball Hamstring Roll-In

Target Muscles: Hamstrings, Gluteus Maximus, Core

Lie on the floor with arms out by your sides. Place both feet atop a stability ball. Engage your core and form a bridge with your midsection by raising your bottom off the floor. Hold this bridge while you bend your knees and use your feet to roll the ball toward your buttocks. Slowly extend your legs, rolling the ball away from your bottom. This is one rep.

Do 10–12 reps.

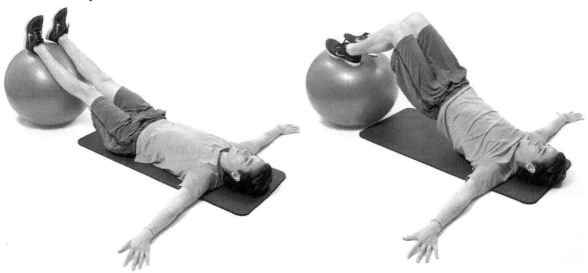

5. Stability Ball Back Extension

Target Muscles: Erector Spinae, Multifidus, Gluteus Maximus

Lie with your stomach on a stability ball and your feet planted wide behind you on the floor. Place your hands by your ears. Slowly extend your back by lifting your torso. Lift until your body makes a diagonal line from your shoulders to your feet. Do not hyperextend your back. Slowly return to the starting position. That's one rep.

Do 10–12 reps.

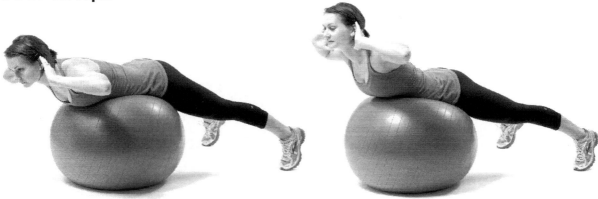

6. Three-Position Calf Raises

Target Muscles: Calves

Holding dumbbells by your sides, step on two weight plates so that just the ball of each foot is on a plate. (You can also do this on the floor without plates.) Both feet should be in a neutral position (facing forward). Slowly lift up on your toes as high as you can, and then slowly lower your heels back to the floor. That's one rep.

Do 10–12 reps.

Repeat with feet facing inward for 10 to 12 reps. Next, repeat with feet facing outward for 10 to 12 reps.

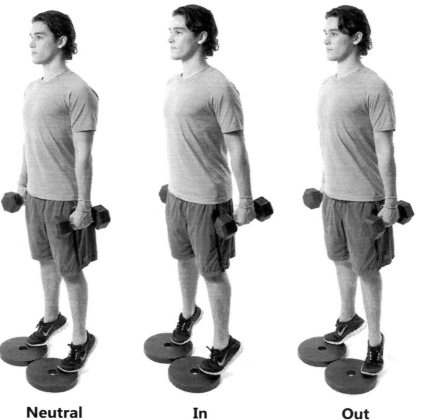

Neutral   **In**   **Out**

Lower Body/Core Workout **INTERMEDIATE**

7. Knee Tuck

Target Muscles: Rectus Abdominis, Internal and External Obliques

Begin in a push-up position with each hand gripping a dumbbell and both legs fully extended behind you and just your toes on the floor. Keeping a neutral spine, move the right knee forward toward the left elbow and rotate the leg under your torso. Return your right leg to the starting position. That's one rep. Repeat with the left leg, moving it toward the right elbow and rotating the left leg under your torso. Continue alternating in this fashion for 30 seconds.

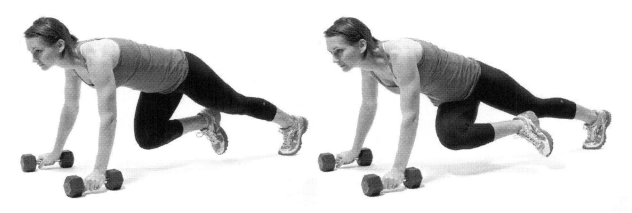

8. Dumbbell Hip-Up

Target Muscles: Gluteus Medius

Holding light dumbbells, stand on the edge of a step so that your left foot is on the step and your right foot is hovering above the floor. Slowly lower your right hip until your right foot moves below the horizon of the step. That's one rep.

Do 10–12 reps.

Face in the opposite direction and repeat with the right foot on the step to work the right gluteus medius. You can do this with or without weights.

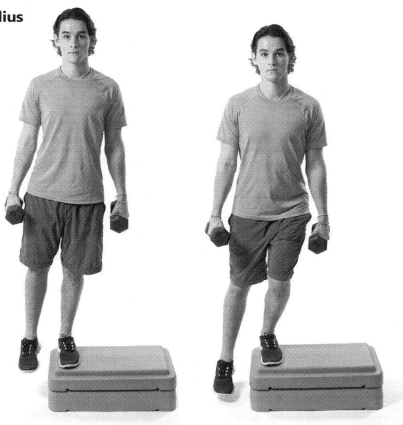

9. Dumbbell Crunch-and-Press
Target Muscles: Rectus Abdominis, Pecs, Triceps, Deltoids

Holding the heads of a dumbbell with your hands, sit on a stability ball. Roll out until the small of your back is resting on the ball. Engage your core and crunch forward as you press the dumbbell straight up above your chest. Slowly lower the dumbbell as you return to the start position. That's one rep.

Do 10–12 reps.

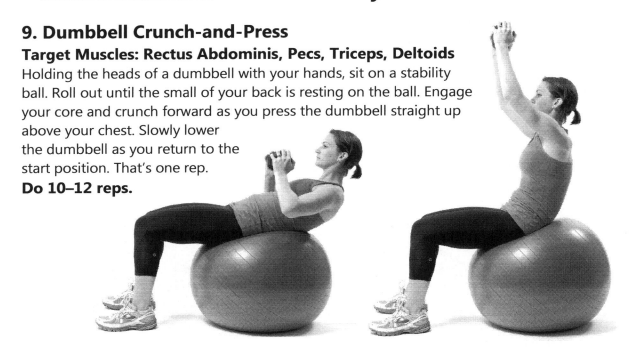

10. Cone Touch
Target Muscles: Quads, Hamstrings, Glutes, Leg-Stabilizer Muscles

Place a cone on the floor two to three feet in front of you. Stand on your right leg with arms at your sides. Lean forward, push your hips back, and extend your left leg behind you, keeping your back straight. Reach out and down with your right hand and try to touch the cone. Return to the starting position without touching your left foot to the floor. That's one rep.

Do 10–12 reps. Repeat standing on your left leg and reaching for the cone with your left hand.

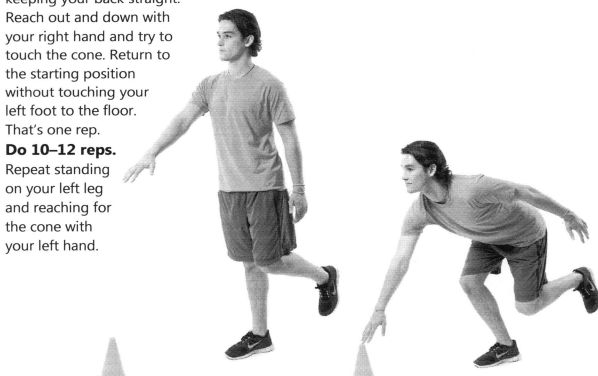

Lower Body/Core Workout INTERMEDIATE

11. Stability Ball Tiger Plank
Target Muscles: Traps, Lats, Erector Spinae, Multifidus, Hip Extensors, Glutes

Lie prone across a stability ball. Be sure the ball is sized so that your hands and feet touch the floor. Simultaneously raise your right arm and left leg until they are both parallel with the floor. Hold for a count of two, then return your arm and leg to the starting position and repeat with the left arm and right leg. Continue alternating opposite arm and leg raises for 30 seconds.

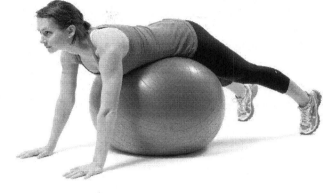

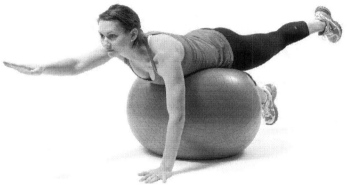

12. Dumbbell Burpee
Target Muscles: Hamstrings, Glutes, Quads

Place a pair of dumbbells on the floor in front of you. Bend down and grip the dumbbells. Engage your core. With your weight on your arms, simultaneously thrust both feet behind you until your legs are fully extended. You should be in a basic push-up position. Quickly return both feet to the original squat position. Release the dumbbells and jump explosively straight up. That's one rep. Upon landing, bend down, grip the dumbbells, and repeat.

Do 10–12 reps.

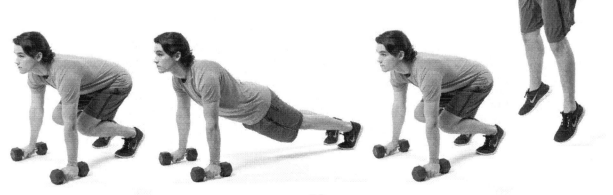

ADVANCED Lower Body/Core Workout

1. Cross-Leg Crunch

Target Muscles: Rectus Abdominis, Internal and External Obliques

Lie on the floor with your knees bent. Cross your left leg over your right knee. Lift your right foot off the floor. Put your right hand beside your right ear. To begin the exercise, engage your core and crunch forward, bringing your right elbow toward your left knee. Your legs should remain still. Lower your torso back to the floor. That's one rep.

Do 12–15 reps.

Repeat with the right leg crossed and left hand by the left ear.

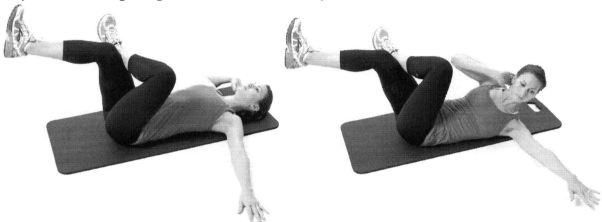

2. Dumbbell Front–Back Lunge

Target Muscles: Quads, Hamstrings, Glutes, Leg-Stabilizer Muscles

Stand tall while holding a light dumbbell at each side. Lunge forward with your right leg. Lower your hips until your upper right leg is parallel with the floor (figure 1). Make sure your knee is in line with or behind your toes. Your back should be straight and not bending at the waist. Balancing on your left leg, lift your right foot off the floor as you return to a standing position and immediately place it on the floor two to three feet behind you (figures 2 and 3). Lower your hips until the calf of your right leg is parallel with the floor. That's one rep.

Do 6–8 reps.

Repeat with the other side.

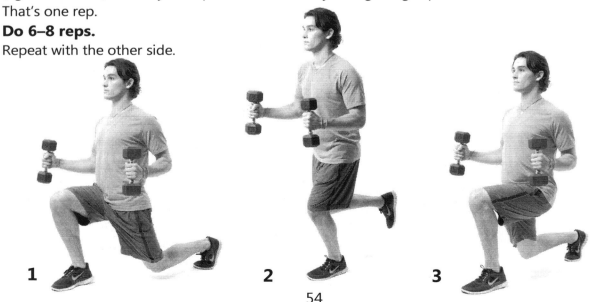

1   2   3

Lower Body/Core Workout <u>ADVANCED</u>

3. Reverse Crunch with 45-Degree Dumbbell Hold
Target Muscles: Rectus Abdominis, Deltoids

Lie on the floor. Holding a dumbbell in each hand with your arms fully extended, slowly lower both arms behind your head until they are at about 45 degrees. Engage your core, then lift your feet as you bend your knees to 90 degrees. Continue pulling your knees toward your chest until your bottom is a few inches off the floor. Slowly return your bottom to the floor. That's one rep.

Do 12–15 reps.

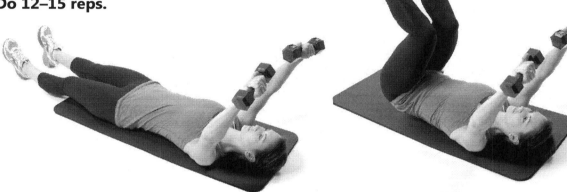

4. Eccentric Single-Leg Hamstring Slide-Out
Target Muscles: Hamstrings, Core

Lie back on the floor. Bend both knees, keeping your feet on the floor. Place a Gliding Disc* underneath your left foot. Lift the right foot and fully extend the right leg. Engage your core as you lift your bottom off the floor into a bridge. While maintaining this bridge, slowly slide your left foot out along the floor. Continue extending the left leg until you're no longer able to maintain the bridge and your bottom drops to the floor. That's one rep.

Do 12–15 reps.

Repeat with the left leg raised and the right foot on the disc. Paper plates or furniture movers also work well on hard or carpeted surfaces.

*Gliding Discs can be purchased at www.power-systems.com.

ADVANCED Lower Body/Core Workout

5. Stability Ball Reverse Hyper
Target Muscles: Gluteus Maximus, Hamstrings, Erector Spinae

Lie prone across a stability ball. Roll out on the ball until your hands are resting on the floor. Raise both legs by extending the hips until the legs are in line with your back. Lower your legs back to the floor. That's one rep.

Do 12–15 reps.

This should be a controlled movement. Do not push off the floor with your feet—lift with your hips.

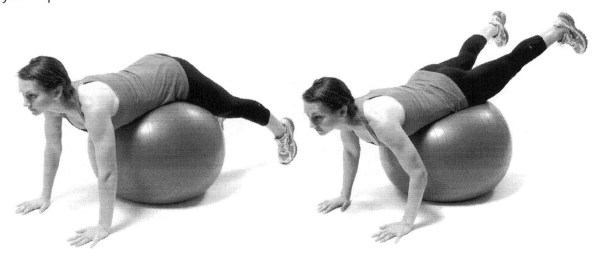

6. Single-Leg Calf Raise
Target Muscles: Calves, Leg-Stabilizer Muscles

Hold a dumbbell in each hand by your sides. Standing with a tall spine and looking straight ahead, lift your right leg. Keeping your left knee locked, raise your left heel by extending the ankle as high as possible. Lower the heel back to the floor. That's one rep.

Do 12–15 reps.

If balance is an issue, hold only one dumbbell and place your free hand on a wall for support.

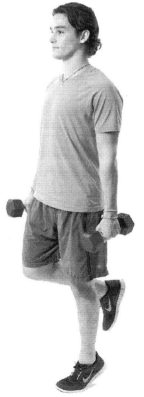

Lower Body/Core Workout <u>**ADVANCED**</u>

7. Knee Drive Plank on Stability Ball
Target Muscles: Rectus Abdominis

Start in an incline plank position on a stability ball. Your arms should be fully extended. Your body should be a diagonal line from your shoulders to heels. Engage your core, and with a slow and controlled movement, lift your right knee up toward your chest. Raise the knee as high as you can, and then slowly lower it back to the floor. Repeat with the left leg. Continue alternating lifting each knee for 30 seconds.

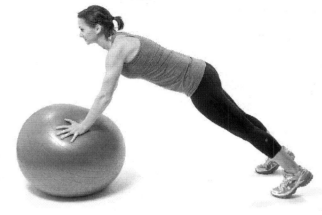

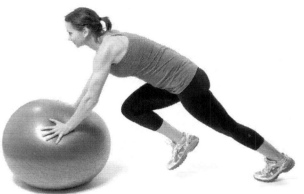

8. Monster Walk
Target Muscles: Hip Abductors, Hip Adductors

Holding each end of an exercise band, step on the center of the band so that your feet are about a foot apart. Stand tall. Keeping the knees locked, move the left leg laterally to the left about 1.5 feet. Keeping the right knee locked, move the right leg inward about halfway toward the left foot. Continue this locked-knee sideways walk to the left for about 10 to 15 feet. Then, facing the same direction, repeat the process side-stepping to the right to work the opposite abductors and adductors. An exercise tube also works well for this exercise.

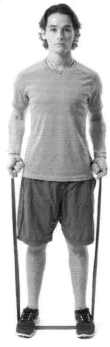

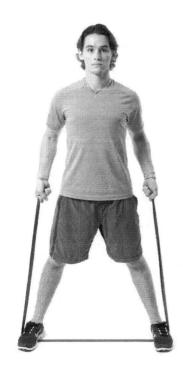

9. Medicine Ball Crunch-and-Press
Target Muscles: Rectus Abdominis, Chest

Lie with your back on the floor. Tuck your feet under heavy dumbbells or the couch, or have someone hold your feet. Hold a medicine ball with both hands at your chest. Engage your core and crunch forward. At the same time, push the medicine ball straight up toward the ceiling. Lower the ball back to your chest as you return your torso to the floor. That's one rep.

Do 12–15 reps.

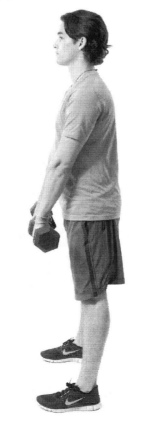

10. Dumbbell Deadlift
Target Muscles: Calves, Hamstrings, Gluteus Maximus, Back

Standing with your feet about shoulder-width apart, hold a dumbbell in each hand with both arms fully extended so the weights rest in front of your thighs. Lower into a squat position by pushing your hips back and bending your knees. Be sure not to round your lower back. With a controlled movement, push yourself back up to the starting position. Pause, and then push yourself back up. That's one rep.

Do 12–15 reps.

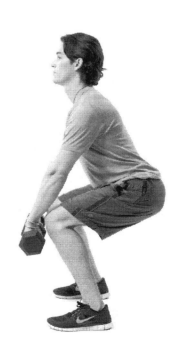

Lower Body/Core Workout **ADVANCED**

11. Front Plank Leg Lift
Target Muscles: Core, Gluteus Maximus

Lie face down on a mat. Engage your core and lift up on your elbows, forearms, and toes. Make sure your elbows are positioned directly underneath your shoulders. Your body should be a straight line from shoulders to heels. Keeping the knee locked, lift and lower your right leg. That's one rep.

Do 12–15 reps.

Repeat with the left leg.

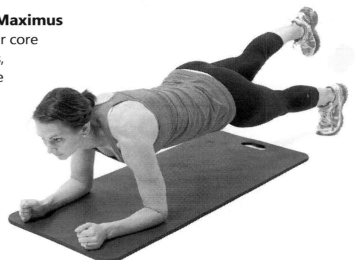

12. Box Jump
Target Muscles: Hamstrings, Gluteus Maximus, Calves, Quads

Stand in front of a sturdy and secure weighted exercise step or box. Start with two stacked steps or a box that's about 12 inches high. Stand about a foot away from the step with your feet shoulder-width apart. Squat down, then jump up with both feet, landing softly on the exercise step. Step down and reposition your feet. That's one rep.

Do 12–15 reps.

Increase the height of the step to increase the intensity of the exercise.

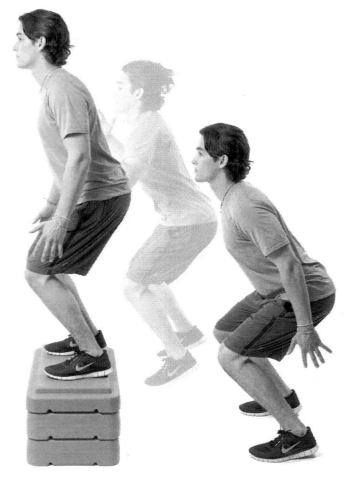

Upper Body/Core Workouts

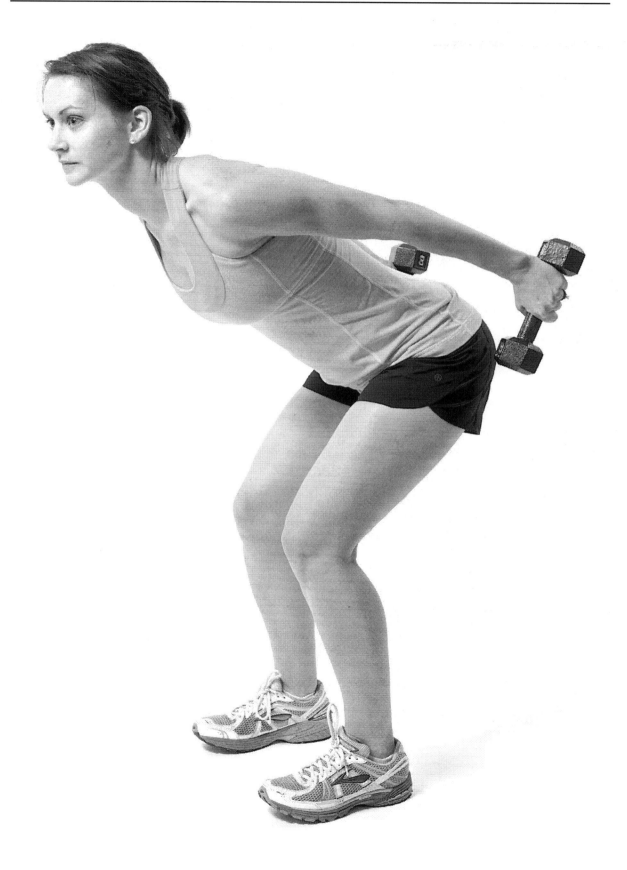

NOVICE Upper Body/Core Workout

1. Medicine Ball Russian Twist (Feet on Floor)
Target Muscles: Rectus Abdominis, Internal and External Obliques

Sit on your bottom with your knees bent and feet flat on the floor. Sit tall and engage your core. Holding a medicine ball with both hands and looking straight ahead, move the ball as far as you can to the right, then swing it back across your torso as far as you can to the left. Control the swing using your obliques to pull the ball from side to side. Continue this back-and-forth motion for 30 seconds.

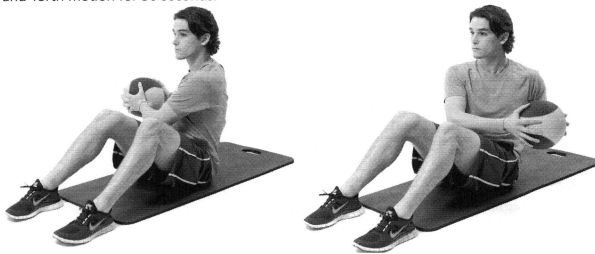

2. Resistance Tube Biceps Curl
Target Muscles: Biceps

Grasp the handles of a resistance tube. Step on the middle of the tube with both feet. Stand up straight with your hands resting at your sides. Bend your elbows, raising both hands toward your shoulders, then slowly lower both hands back to the starting position. That's one rep.

Do 8–10 reps.

To increase tension, position your feet farther apart on the tube. To decrease tension, bring the feet closer together or step on the tube with only one foot.

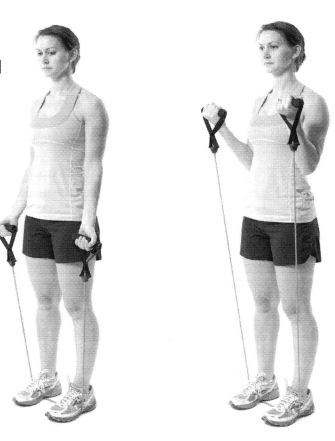

Upper Body/Core Workout <u>**NOVICE**</u>

3. Big Circle

Target Muscles: Core, Rotator Cuffs, Lats

Stand tall with your feet shoulder-width apart. Hold a medicine ball with both hands in front of your waist, arms fully extended. Keeping your elbows straight, move the ball in a clockwise direction, making a big circle back to the starting position. That's one rep.

Do 8–10 reps.

Repeat, moving the ball counterclockwise.

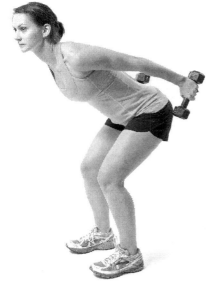

4. Dumbbell Hammer Curl Kickback

Target Muscles: Triceps, Biceps

In each hand, hold a dumbbell with a neutral grip (palms facing inward) by your sides. Stand tall with your feet shoulder-width apart. Bend your knees slightly. Keeping your back flat, bend forward at the waist. Moving just your lower arms, bring the dumbbells up to your shoulders. This is the starting position. With a controlled movement, lower the dumbbells and push your arms back until both arms are fully extended. With a controlled movement, return your arms to the starting position. That's one rep.

Do 8–10 reps.

Be careful not to swing the dumbbells. Decrease the weight if you're unable to fully extend your arms.

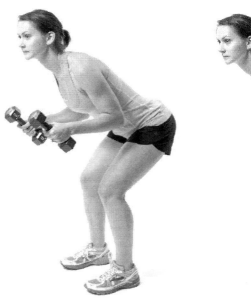

5. Stability Ball Crunch

Target Muscles: Rectus Abdominis

Sit on a stability ball and roll out until the small of your back is resting on the ball. Position your hands beside your ears. Do not pull on your neck. If this is a temptation, place your arms across your chest instead. Engage your core and exhale as you lift your torso forward. Using a controlled movement, lower your torso back to the starting position. That's one rep.

Do 8–10 reps.

Avoid pushing back with your feet and rocking back on your knees. Only your torso moves during this exercise. Keep your knees bent at 90 degrees throughout the exercise.

6. Dumbbell Chest Press

Target Muscles: Pecs, Triceps

Lie on a weight bench. Hold a dumbbell in each hand with both arms fully extended above your chest. Bend both arms at the elbow and slowly lower the dumbbells until they are just above your chest. Fully extend both arms, returning the dumbbells to the start position. That's one rep.

Do 8–10 reps.

If you do not have a weight bench, you can perform this exercise while lying on the floor.

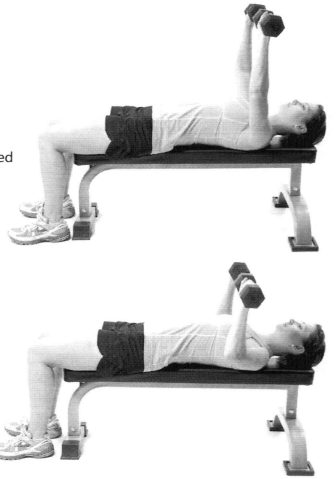

Upper Body/Core Workout

7. Low/High Medicine Ball Chop
Target Muscles: Internal and External Obliques, Lats

Holding a medicine ball to the left of your hip, position your feet shoulder-width apart and bend your knees slightly. Looking straight ahead, raise the ball diagonally, moving your hands from your left hip to above your right shoulder. As you raise the ball, extend your legs. Lower the ball back to the left side of your hip as you bend your knees. That's one rep.

Do 8–10 reps.

Repeat, starting at the right side of the hip and raising the ball over your left shoulder.

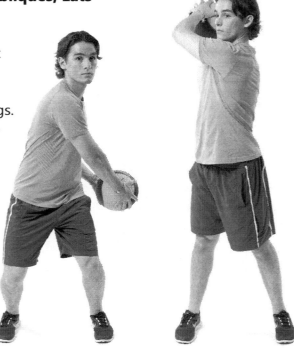

8. Stability Ball Dumbbell T-Raise
Target Muscles: Delts, Upper Back, Triceps

Lie prone across a stability ball with your toes firmly planted behind you. Grasp a light dumbbell in each hand so that your palms are facing you. Simultaneously raise both arms out to the side, lifting the dumbbells until both arms are parallel with the floor. Slowly lower both arms, returning the dumbbells to the start position. That's one rep.

Do 8–10 reps.

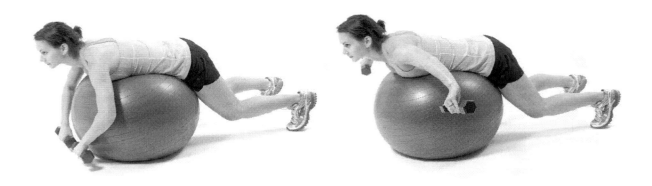

9. Dumbbell Scissor Kicks

Target Muscles: Rectus Abdominis, Hip Abductors and Adductors

Lie with your back on the floor. Grasp the heads of a dumbbell and hold it just above your chest. With your shoulders raised off the floor, lift both feet about six inches. Spread your legs apart, and then bring them back to center until they cross. Continue this back-and-forth scissors motion for 30 seconds.

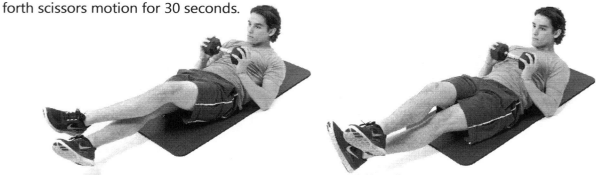

10. Resistance Tube Front Raise/Side Raise

Target Muscles: Front and Middle Delts

Grasp the handles of a resistance tube. Step on the center of the tube with both feet. Stand upright with your hands resting in front of your thighs. Keeping your arms fully extended, raise both arms straight up in front of you until they're parallel with the floor. Lower your arms back to your thighs. Then, still keeping your arms fully extended, raise both arms out to the side until they're both parallel with the floor. Lower your arms to the starting position. That's one rep.

Do 8–10 reps.

For more resistance, position your feet wider apart. For less resistance, bring your feet closer together or step on the tube with just one foot.

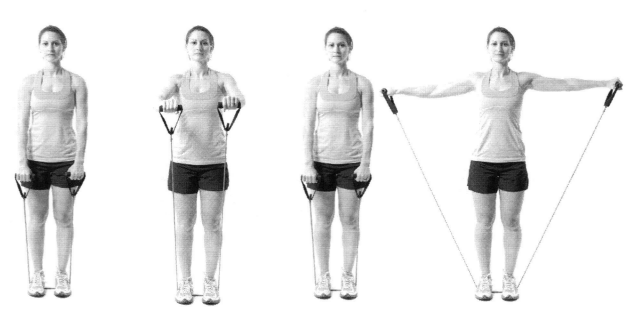

Upper Body/Core Workout **NOVICE**

11. 30-Second Front Plank
Target Muscles: Erector Spinae, Rectus Abdominis, Transverse Abdominis

Lie face down on the floor so that your forearms are on the floor under your chest. Engage your core and lift your body so that only your forearms, elbows, and toes are touching the floor. Your body should be a straight line from your shoulders to your toes. Make sure your midsection does not arch up or sag. Also make sure that your elbows are positioned directly under your shoulders. Hold this position for 30 seconds.

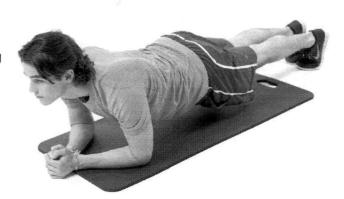

12. Single-Arm Dumbbell Row
Target Muscles: Lats, Trapezius, Rear Delts, Biceps

Extend your left leg behind you, and then lean forward on your right leg, resting your right hand on your thigh. Look straight ahead and keep your back flat. Hold a dumbbell in your left hand with the palm facing in. Raise the dumbbell vertically alongside your torso. Raise your elbow as high as you can before lowering the dumbbell back to the starting position. That's one rep.

Do 8–10 reps.

Repeat with the other side.

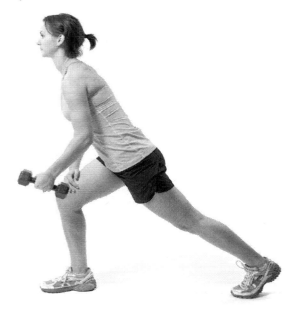
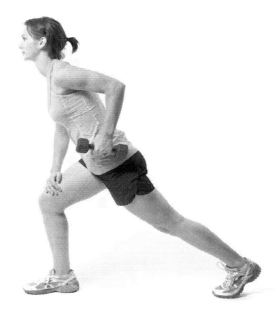

INTERMEDIATE Upper Body/Core Workout

1. Medicine Ball Russian Twist (Feet Lifted)
Target Muscles: Rectus Abdominis, Internal and External Obliques

Grasp a medicine ball and sit on a mat with your knees bent and feet on the floor. Engage your core, lift your feet, and lean back 45 degrees. Looking straight ahead, move the ball as far as you can to the right, then swing it back across your torso as far as you can to the left. Control the swing using your obliques to pull the ball from side to side. Continue this back-and-forth motion for 30 seconds.

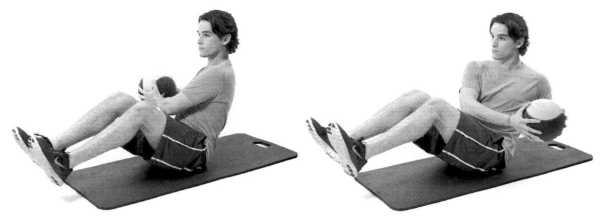

2. Dumbbell Curl-and-Press
Target Muscles: Biceps, Deltoids

Stand holding dumbbells at thigh level (palms facing away). Curl the dumbbells up toward your shoulders. At the shoulders, turn the dumbbells so your palms are facing out. Press both dumbbells overhead until your arms are fully extended. Carefully lower the dumbbells back to your shoulders. Turn the dumbbells so that your palms are facing in. Lower the dumbbells back to your thighs. That's one rep.

Do 10–12 reps.

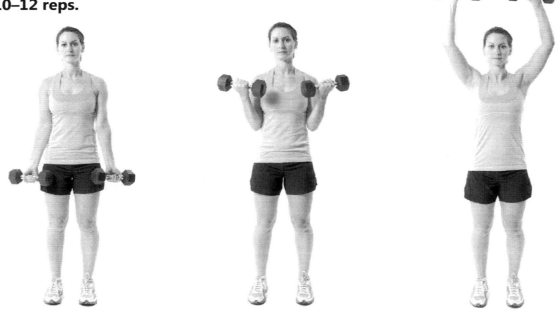

3. Stability Ball Side Crunch
Target Muscles: Internal and External Obliques

Lie on your left side on a stability ball. Spread your legs wide and plant your feet on the floor for a stable base. Place your hands by your ears. Engage your obliques to lift your torso off the ball. Slowly return your torso back to the ball. That's one rep.

Do 10–12 reps.

Repeat with your right side lying on the ball.

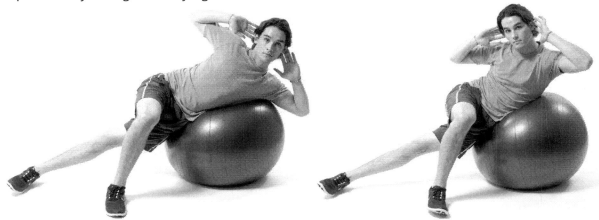

4. Resistance Tube Overhead Triceps Extension
Target Muscles: Triceps

Grasp the resistance tube handles. Step on the tube with your left foot. Let your left arm hang down by your side while still holding the resistance tube handle. Using your right hand, lift the other end of the resistance tube up behind your body until your elbow is pointing straight up to the ceiling. This is the starting position. From this position, raise the forearm of your right arm until your arm is fully extended. The upper arm should remain still during this movement. Slowly lower your forearm back to the starting position. That's one rep.

Do 10–12 reps.

Repeat with your left arm. If your resistance tube is too short to hold with the opposite hand, you can drop the handle and secure it in place with your foot firmly planted on the resistance tube.

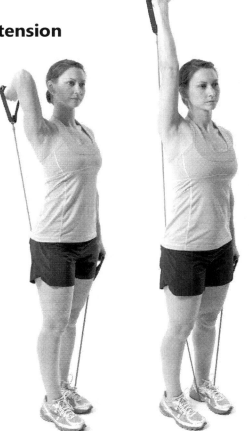

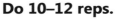

5. Medicine Ball Knee-Up Crunch

Target Muscles: Rectus Abdominis, Delts, Lats, Rotator Cuffs, Hip Flexors

Lie on the floor on your back. Place a medicine ball above the top of your head. Reach above your head with both arms and grasp the ball. Keeping your arms fully extended, lift your shoulders off the mat and bring the ball over your head. At the same time that you're lifting your shoulders, lift your right foot off the floor, bend your knee and raise it toward your chest. Continue pulling the ball over your head until it reaches just past your knee. Keeping your arms fully extended, slowly lower the ball to the floor just above your head while also returning your right leg to the floor. That's one rep. Alternate knees each time your crunch forward with the ball.

Do 10–12 reps.

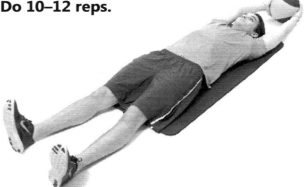

6. Stability Ball Dumbbell Pec Fly

Target Muscles: Pecs, Core

Lie back on a stability ball. Roll out on your back until your head and neck are supported on the ball. Holding a dumbbell in each hand with a neutral grip (palms facing each other), fully extend your arms above your chest. This is the starting position. Using a controlled movement, lower your arms out to the sides of your chest as if you're undoing a bear hug. Your arms should be slightly bent at the elbow. Return the dumbbells back above your chest. That's one rep.

Do 10–12 reps.

The stability ball requires engagement of the core to keep your balance. As you acclimate to the balance elements, try using lighter weights than you would use if performing this exercise on a bench.

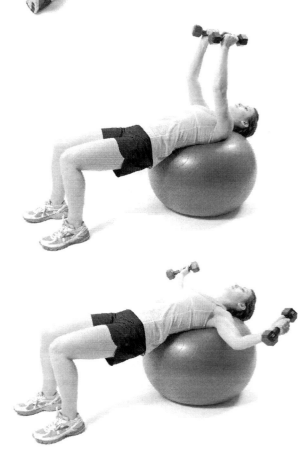

Upper Body/Core Workout <u>**INTERMEDIATE**</u>

7. Side Plank-Up
Target Muscles: Internal and External Obliques, Rectus Abdominis, Transverse Abdominis

Lie on your right side with your legs fully extended and your feet stacked. Prop your torso up on your right elbow. Make sure your elbow is directly underneath your shoulder. Put your left hand on your hip. Engage your core and raise your hips off the floor until your body creates a diagonal line from your shoulders to your feet. Using a controlled movement, lower your hips back to the floor. That's one rep.

Do 10–12 reps.

Repeat on your left side.

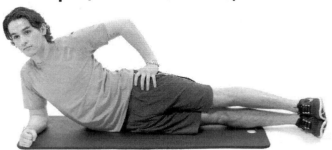

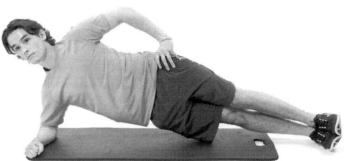

8. Seated Reverse Dumbbell Fly
Target Muscles: Middle and Upper Back, Rear Deltoids, Rotator Cuffs

Grasp a pair of light dumbbells and sit on the end of a weight bench. Lean forward about 45 degrees, positioning the dumbbells just below your thighs. Keep a flat back (don't round your shoulders) and a slight bend at the elbow. Engage your upper-back muscles and, without moving your torso, raise your elbows until they are parallel with the floor. Lower the dumbbells back to the start position. That's one rep.

Do 10–12 reps.

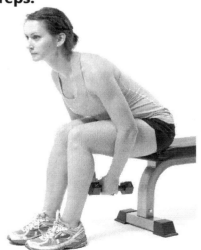

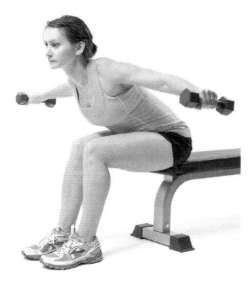

9. Single-Leg Pull-In
Target Muscles: Rectus Abdominis, Hip Flexors

Lie on the floor and tuck your hands under the small of your back. Engage your core, then lift both feet just a few inches off the floor. While keeping the left leg fully extended, bend the right knee and pull it toward your torso. Fully extend the right leg back to the start position. That's one rep.

Do 10–12 reps.

Repeat with the left leg.

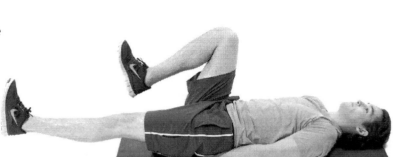

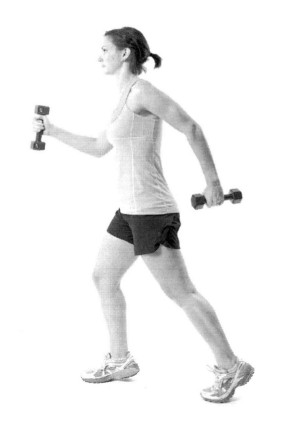

10. Dumbbell Runner Swing
Target Muscles: Deltoids, Lats, Core

Stand tall with a light dumbbell in each hand (neutral grip). Assume a runner's stance with one foot slightly ahead of the other, knees slightly bent. Remaining stationary, begin alternately swinging the dumbbells beside your torso. The front dumbbell should reach about chest or shoulder level, and the rear dumbbell should reach just past your buttocks at waist level. Continue this alternating exaggerated motion for 30 seconds.

Upper Body/Core Workout

11. Stability Ball Roll-Out
Target Muscles: Rectus Abdominis, Erector Spinae

Kneel upright on an exercise mat. Position your hands with palms touching on a stability ball. Engage your core, then roll the ball forward until only your forearms and elbows are on the ball. Drop your hips as you roll forward until your body is a straight plank from your shoulders to your knees. To complete the motion, use your core muscles to roll back on the ball, pulling your torso back to the starting position. That's one rep.

Do 10–12 reps.

When you roll out, if your chest is on the ball, try positioning your hands farther down on the ball before rolling out.

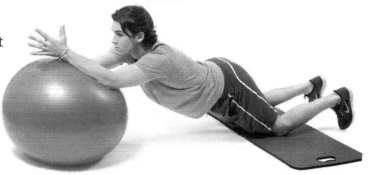

12. Rear Deltoid Dumbbell Raise
Target Muscles: Rear Deltoids, Rotator Cuffs

Lie on your right side atop a stability ball so that your right hand and both feet are on the floor. Your body should be straight. The feet can be fanned out for more stability if needed. Grasp a light dumbbell in your left hand. Starting at the floor, begin raising the dumbbell until your arm is perpendicular with your body. Be careful not to over-rotate your arm. Using a controlled motion, slowly lower the dumbbell back to the floor. That's one rep.

Do 10–12 reps.

Repeat on your left side, raising the dumbbell with your right hand.

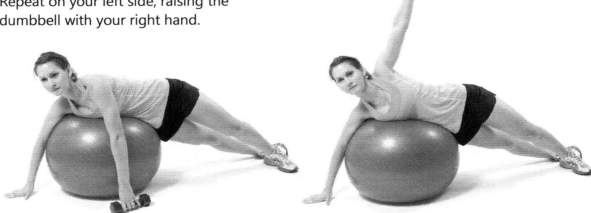

ADVANCED Upper Body/Core Workout

1. Pendulum

Target Muscles: Rectus Abdominis, Internal and External Obliques

Lie on your back with your arms stretched out to both sides. Raise both legs straight up until they are perpendicular with the floor. Using a controlled movement and with feet together, lower both legs to the right as close to the floor as possible, keeping your shoulders on the floor. Use your core muscles to pull your legs back up to center and over to the left side as close to the floor as possible. This is one rep.

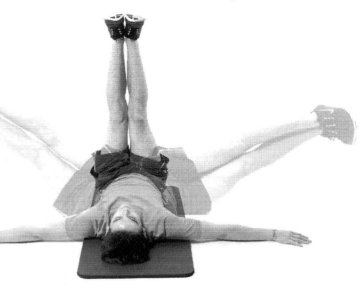

Do 12–15 reps.

If needed, grip heavy dumbbells as anchor weights to help keep your shoulders from lifting off the floor.

2. Static Biceps Curl

Target Muscles: Biceps

Grasp a dumbbell in each hand. Stand tall, and with palms facing out, fully extend your arms so the dumbbells are resting in front of your thighs. Raise the dumbbell in the left hand until your elbow makes a 90-degree angle. While keeping the left arm at 90 degrees, curl the dumbbell in the right arm up to your right shoulder. That's one rep.

Do 12–15 reps.

Repeat by holding the right arm at 90 degrees and curling the dumbbell in your left hand. (If desired, you can add a balance element to this exercise by standing on a balance disk.)

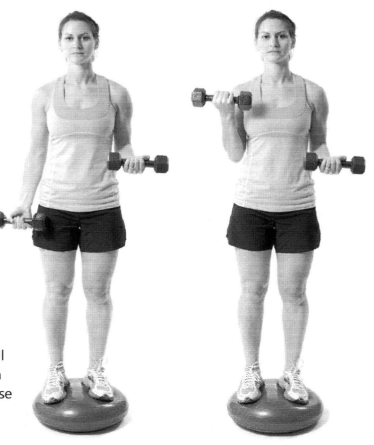

Upper Body/Core Workout <u>**ADVANCED**</u>

3. Stability Ball Jackknife with Pike

Target Muscles: Rectus Abdominis, Erector Spinae

Rest your forearms and elbows on a bench. Place both feet behind you atop a stability ball so that your shins are resting on the ball. Engage your core and pull your knees in toward your chest. Keeping the core engaged, push your feet back on the ball, returning your legs to the start position. That's one rep.

Do 12–15 reps.

For a more advanced version, add a pike to the movement by lifting the hips up as you pull your knees toward your chest.

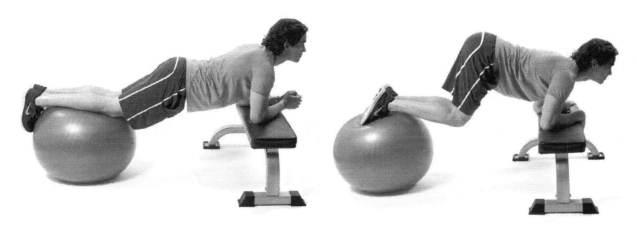

4. Lying Stability Ball Triceps Extension

Target Muscles: Triceps

Grasp a pair of dumbbells and sit on a stability ball. Roll out on the ball until your head and neck are supported on the ball. Hold the dumbbells directly above your chest with your arms fully extended. Using a controlled motion, bend your elbows and lower both dumbbells, stopping when they're just past your ears. Raise both dumbbells until your arms are fully extended. That's one rep.

Do 12–15 reps.

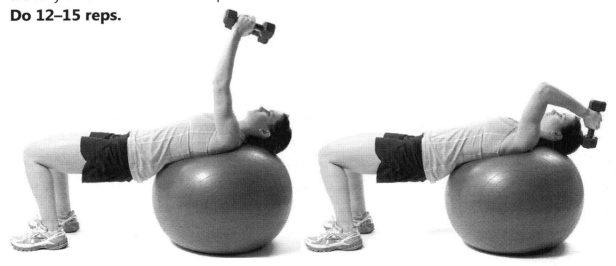

5. Medicine Ball Double Crunch

Target Muscles: Rectus Abdominis, Hip Adductors

Lie on your back. Place a medicine ball between your knees. Hold the ball in place by squeezing your adductor (inner thigh) muscles together. Hold another medicine ball with both hands at your chest. Crunch forward, lifting your shoulders off the floor and keeping the ball at your chest while at the same time lifting your feet off the floor and bringing your knees toward your chest. Return your shoulders and feet to the floor. That's one rep.

Do 12–15 reps.

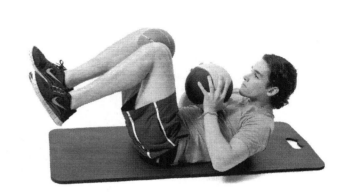

6. Offset Medicine Ball Push-Up

Target Muscles: Pecs, Triceps

From a standard push-up position, place one hand atop a medicine ball. Engage your core, and then bend at the elbow, lowering your chest toward the floor. Lower as far as you can, then push back up. That's one rep. Roll the ball to the other hand before completing the next rep.

Do 12–16 reps.

You can also perform this exercise using a modified push-up position with your knees on the floor. In this position, be sure to lower your hips so that your body forms a straight line from your knees to your shoulders.

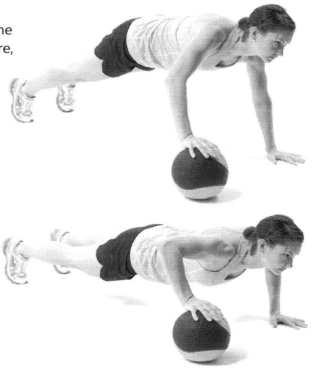

Upper Body/Core Workout **ADVANCED**

7. Side Plank with Dumbbell Rotation
Target Muscles: Internal and External Obliques, Rear Delts, Rectus Abdominis

Lie on your right side with your legs fully extended and your feet stacked. Prop your torso up on your right elbow. Make sure your elbow is directly underneath your shoulder. Grasp a light dumbbell in your left hand. Start with the dumbbell slightly underneath the right side of your torso. Rotate the left arm up and out until your arm is fully extended and perpendicular to your body. Control the movement, being careful not to over-rotate your arm. Slowly lower the dumbbell, following the same pathway back underneath your torso. That's one rep.

Do 12–15 reps.

Repeat on your left side, rotating the dumbbell with your right hand.

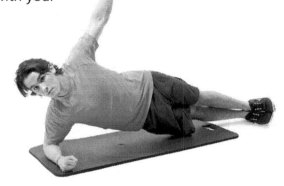

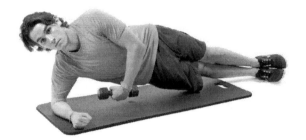

8. Standing Dumbbell T-Raise
Target Muscles: Front and Rear Delts, Rotator Cuffs, Upper Back

Stand tall while holding light dumbbells in front of your thighs, palms facing your thighs. Keeping your elbows locked, raise your arms in front of you until they are parallel with the floor. Keeping the dumbbells at this same level and your elbows locked, move your arms laterally until you've formed a T with your body. Next, bring the dumbbells back to the front of your torso, and slowly lower them back to the starting position. That's one rep.

Do 12–15 reps.

To increase the difficulty level, stand on a balance disk.

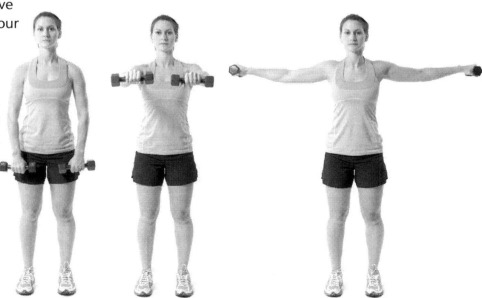

9. Dumbbell Leg Lift
Target Muscles: Rectus Abdominis, Hip Adductors

Lie on the floor with a lightweight dumbbell between your feet. Tuck your hands under the small of your back for support. Engage your core and squeeze your feet together to secure the dumbbell. Lift your legs about a foot off the floor, keeping the dumbbell between your feet. Lower your feet until they're about one inch off the floor. That's one rep.
Do 12–15 reps.

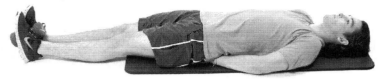

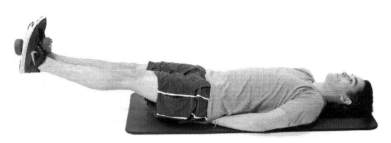

10. Single-Foot Stability Ball Dumbbell Shoulder Press
Target Muscles: Rectus Abdominis, Hip Adductors

Grasp a pair of dumbbells and sit on top of a stability ball. Sit up straight with a tall spine. Position the dumbbells at shoulder level with palms facing away from you. Engage your core and lift your right foot a few inches off the floor. Keeping the foot off the floor, press the dumbbells straight up until your arms are fully extended. Lower the dumbbells back to shoulder level. That's one rep.

Do 12–15 reps.

Do half of the reps with the right foot raised and half with the left foot raised. Due to the added stability element of sitting on the ball with one foot lifted, use lighter dumbbells than you would use if performing a shoulder press seated on a bench.

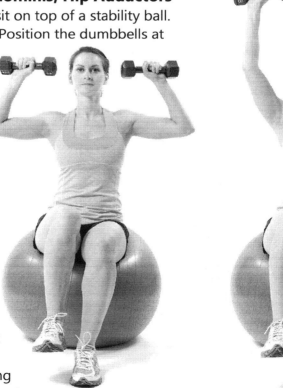

11. Cycling Russian Twist

Target Muscles: Internal and External Obliques, Rectus Abdominis, Hip Flexors

Sit on a mat. Raise your feet a few inches off the floor and lean back about 45 degrees. Extend your arms in front of your torso and bring your hands together (palms facing each other). Pull your right knee toward your chest and twist your torso, swinging your hands (arms fully extended) to the outside of your right knee. Then pull in the left knee while fully extending the right knee. Twist your torso to the left, swinging your hands to the outside of the left knee. Continue this cycling/twisting motion for 30 seconds.

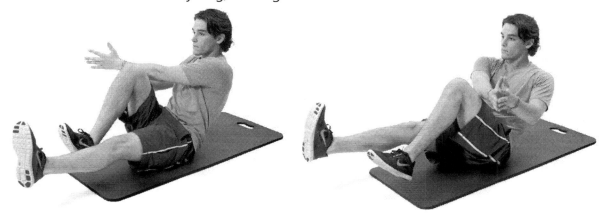

12. Bent-Over Row with Back Extension

Target Muscles: Lats, Erector Spinae

Grasp a pair of dumbbells and stand with your feet about shoulder-width apart. Lean forward at the waist until your torso is parallel with the floor. Your knees should be slightly bent. Extend your arms so the dumbbells rest at or slightly below your knees. This is the starting position. Pull the dumbbells up toward the sides of your torso. Keeping the dumbbells at this position, raise your torso to a standing position. That's one rep.

Do 12–15 reps.

To begin the next rep, keep the dumbbells by your rib cage and return to the bent-over position. Lower the dumbbells to knee level.

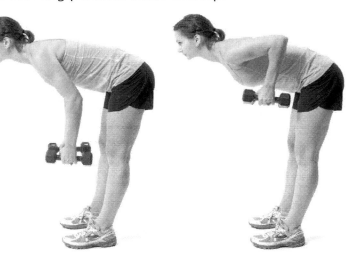

Full-Body Exercises

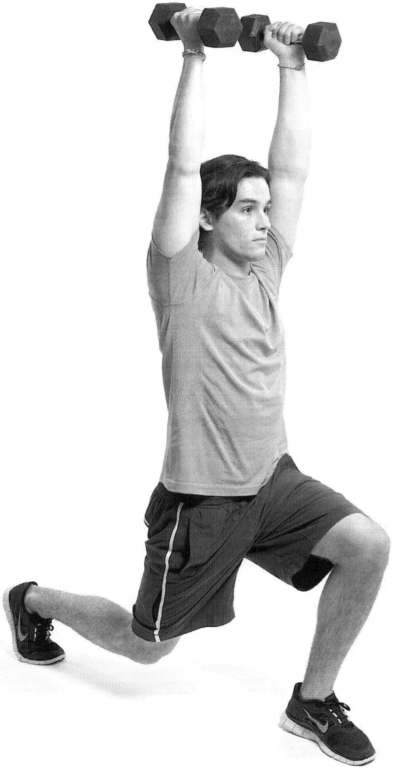

Working multiple muscle groups at the same time is a great way to exercise the body. After all, muscles are rarely ever used in isolation in your everyday activities.

This section contains four multijoint, full-body exercises. Feel free to swap out one of the exercises in the previous upper-body/core or lower-body/core chapters with one of these full-body exercises, or simply add one of the full-body exercises to a workout.

If you're a novice, complete eight to 10 repetitions. Intermediate-level athletes should complete 10 to 12 repetitions. At the advanced level, complete 12 to 15 repetitions.

Don't have time for an entire 12-exercise circuit? No problem. Use one or two of these full-body exercises for a quick quality workout.

Full-Body Exercises

Burpee Dumbbell Press
Target Muscles: Legs, Core, Shoulders

Stand tall holding dumbbells by your sides. Bend at the hips and the waist to lower your body placing the dumbbells on the floor (1). Gripping the dumbbells, kick both feet out behind you creating a diagonal plank (2). Immediately draw your feet back toward your chest so that your feet are beneath you (3). Stand up, raising your arms and pressing the dumbbells overhead (4). That's one rep.

Novice: 8–10 reps. Intermediate: 10–12 reps. Advanced: 12–15 reps.

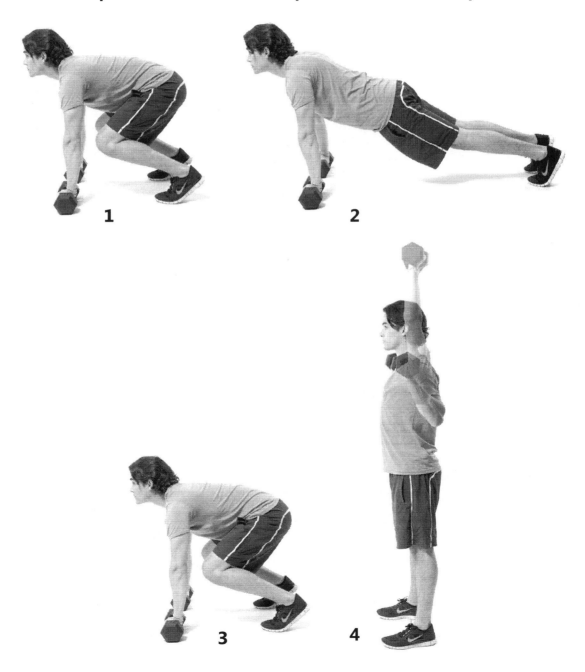

Full-Body Exercises

Dumbbell Push Press with Twist
Target Muscles: Legs, Core, Shoulders

Grasp a pair of dumbbells and stand with your feet about shoulder-width apart. Position the dumbbells at your shoulders with your palms facing in (1). Push your hips back and lower into a squat position, making sure your knees are behind or in line with your toes (2). Explosively push up with your legs while pressing the dumbbells overhead and rotating your torso to the right (3). Lower the dumbbells and bend back into a squat. That's one rep. Alternate twisting your torso to the right and left with each press.

Novice: 8–10 reps. Intermediate: 10–12 reps.
Advanced: 12–15 reps.

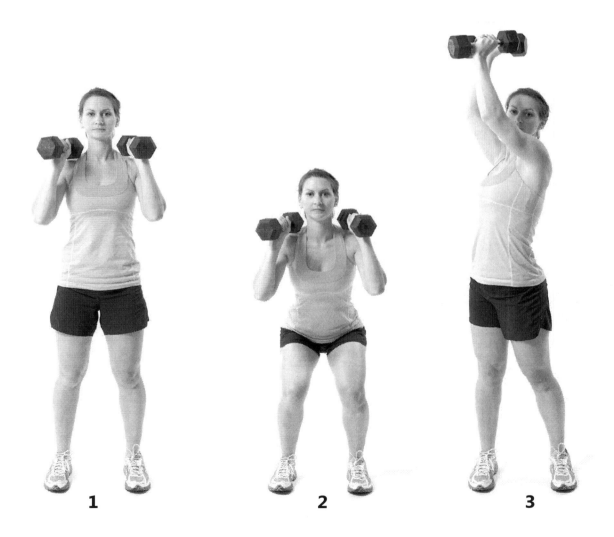

1   2   3

Full-Body Exercises

Dumbbell Lunge, Hammer Curl, Press
Target Muscles: Legs, Core, Biceps, Shoulders

Stand tall, holding a dumbbell at each side. Lunge forward with your right leg while raising the dumbbells (with a neutral grip) toward your shoulders (this is a hammer curl). Once at the shoulders, press the dumbbells overhead, fully extending the arms. Return to the start position by lowering the dumbbells and extending the knees to a standing position. That's one rep. Alternate legs with each rep.

Novice: 8–10 reps.

Intermediate: 10–12 reps.

Advanced: 12–15 reps.

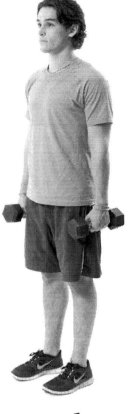

1

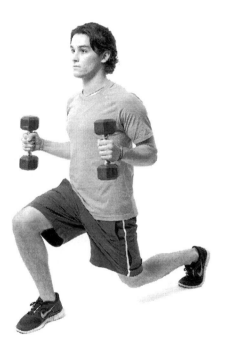

2

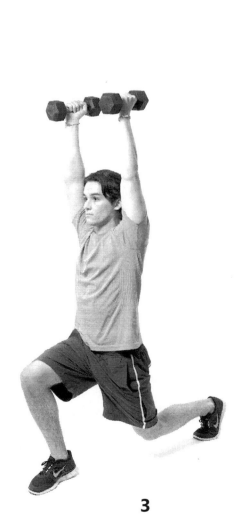

3

Full-Body Exercises

Dumbbell Hammer Squat

Target Muscles: Legs, Core, Biceps

Stand with your feet shoulder-width apart. Hold a dumbbell at each side. Push your hips back and lower into a squat until your thighs are parallel with the floor. While squatting, curl the dumbbells up toward your shoulders, then lower the dumbbells to your sides as you return to a standing position.

Novice: 8–10 reps. Intermediate: 10–12 reps. Advanced: 12–15 reps.

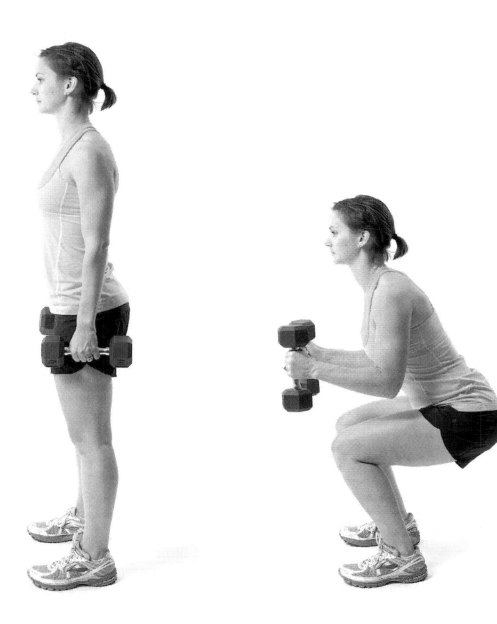

More for the Core

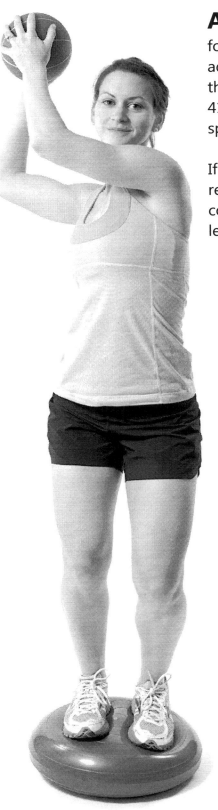

A strong core is a crucial part of good running form. The following eight exercises can be added to or used as alternate core exercises for the lower-body and upper-body circuits (pages 41–79). You can also use them as an extra circuit specifically targeting the core.

If you're a novice, complete eight to 10 repetitions. Intermediate-level athletes should complete 10 to 12 repetitions. At the advanced level, complete 12 to 15 repetitions.

Additional Core Exercises

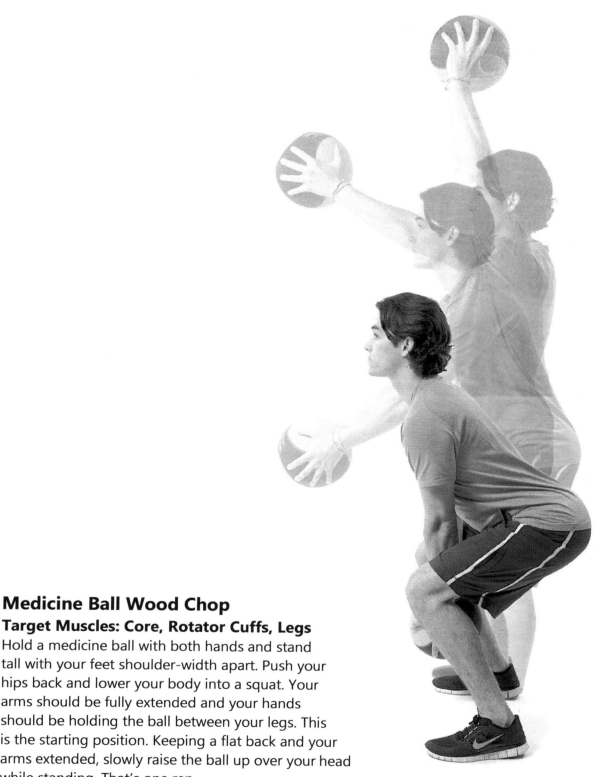

Medicine Ball Wood Chop
Target Muscles: Core, Rotator Cuffs, Legs

Hold a medicine ball with both hands and stand tall with your feet shoulder-width apart. Push your hips back and lower your body into a squat. Your arms should be fully extended and your hands should be holding the ball between your legs. This is the starting position. Keeping a flat back and your arms extended, slowly raise the ball up over your head while standing. That's one rep.

Novice: 8–10 reps. Intermediate: 10–12 reps. Advanced: 12–15 reps.

Additional Core Exercises

Twist, Plop, Grab
Target Muscles: Internal and External Obliques

Sit on an exercise mat with your knees bent and your feet on the floor in front of you. Hold a medicine ball at chest level. This is the starting position.

Twist your torso to the right and place the ball behind your back. After releasing the ball, twist your torso to the left. Reach around with both hands, grab the ball and bring it to center, making one complete revolution around your body. That's one rep.

Novice: 8–10 reps.
Intermediate: 10–12 reps.
Advanced: 12–15 reps.

Do half of the reps in this direction, then reverse direction for the second half.

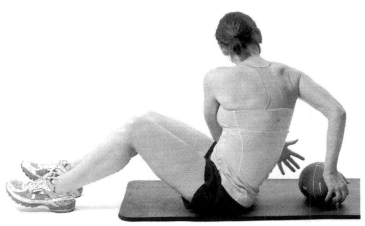

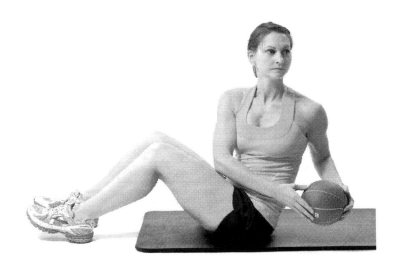

Additional Core Exercises

Side Plank with Leg Adduction

Target Muscles: Internal and External Obliques, Hip Adductors, Erector Spinae, Gluteus Medius, Gluteus Minimus

Lie on your side on an exercise mat. Place a small stability ball between your legs. Lift up on your left elbow and forearm. Place your right hand on your hip. Squeeze your legs together for a two count. That's one rep. Do the desired number of reps while holding the side plank position, then flip and repeat with your right elbow and forearm on the mat and left hand on your hip.

Novice: 8–10 reps. Intermediate: 10–12 reps. Advanced: 12–15 reps.

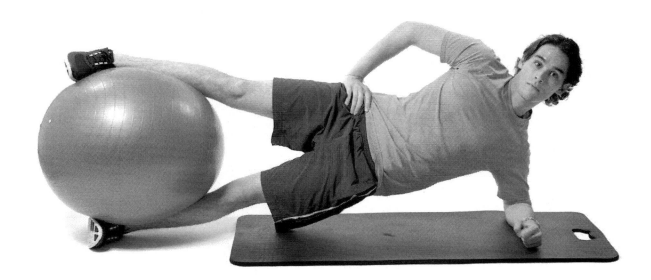

Additional Core Exercises

Low High Chop on Balance Disk
Target Muscles: Internal and External Obliques, Lats, Leg Stabilizers

Grasp a medicine ball and carefully stand on top of a balance disk. Bend your knees slightly and hold the ball at the left side of your hip. Extend your knees while lifting the ball up and over your right shoulder. Lower the ball as you bend your knees and return to the starting position. That's one rep. Do the desired number of reps, then repeat moving the ball from the right side of the hip up and over the left shoulder.

Novice: 8–10 reps. Intermediate: 10–12 reps. Advanced: 12–15 reps.

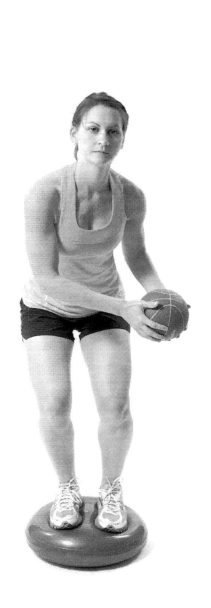
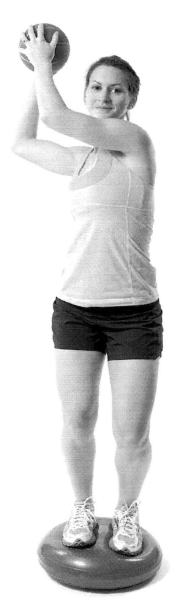

Additional Core Exercises

Medicine Ball Knee-Over

Target Muscles: Internal and External Obliques, Hip Adductors

Sit on an exercise mat and place a medicine ball between your knees. Squeeze your knees together to hold the ball in place. Lie back on the mat and stretch your arms out to the sides. Lift your feet until your calves are parallel with the floor. This is the starting position. Engage your core. With a controlled movement, lower your knees as far to the left as you can without allowing your right shoulder to lift off the mat. Use your obliques to pull knees back to center, then lower them as far to the right as you can without allowing your left shoulder to lift off the mat. That's one rep.

Novice: 8–10 reps.

Intermediate: 10–12 reps.

Advanced: 12–15 reps.

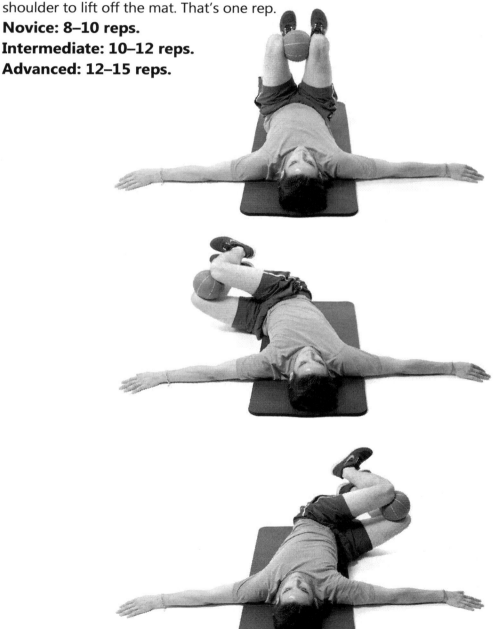

Additional Core Exercises

Side-Lying Knee Crunch
Target Muscles: Rectus Abdominis, Internal and External Obliques

Sit on an exercise mat with your knees bent and feet on the floor. Lie back on the mat. Lean your knees to the left, keeping your shoulders on the floor. Place your hands beside your ears. This is the starting position. Engage your core and crunch forward, lifting your shoulders straight up and off the floor. Return your shoulders to the floor. That's one rep. Do the desired number of reps, and then repeat with your knees leaning to the right.

Novice: 8–10 reps. Intermediate: 10–12 reps. Advanced: 12–15 reps.

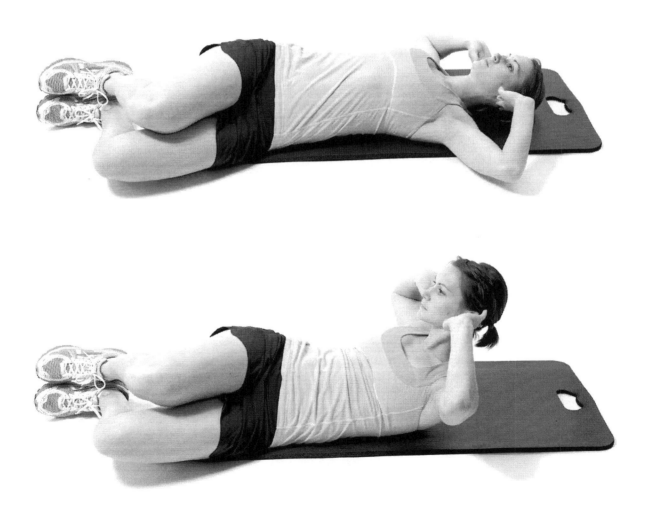

Additional Core Exercises

Standing Russian Twist on Balance Disk
Target Muscles: Internal and External Obliques, Leg Stabilizers

Grasp a medicine ball and carefully stand on a balance disk. Bend your knees slightly. Engage your core and hold the ball out from your torso. Look ahead and twist your torso to the left. Using a controlled movement, twist your torso to the right. That's one rep.

Novice: 8–10 reps. Intermediate: 10–12 reps. Advanced: 12–15 reps.

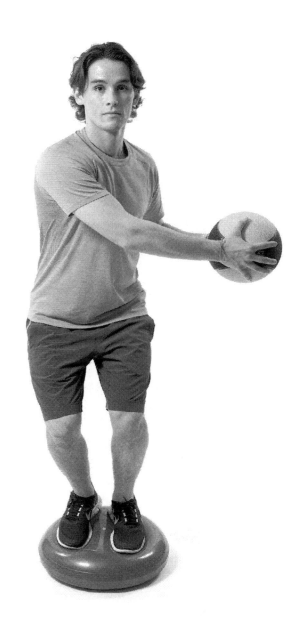

Additional Core Exercises

Dumbbell Drag
Target Muscles: Rectus Abdominis, Rotator Cuffs

Grasp a pair of light dumbbells and lie back on the floor. Raise both legs in the air, feet together. Extend your arms, holding the dumbbells above your chest with a neutral grip. This is the starting position. Slowly lower your arms until they almost touch the floor, and then return them to the starting position. That's one rep.

Novice: 8–10 reps. Intermediate: 10–12 reps. Advanced: 12–15 reps.

To increase the intensity of this exercise, lower your legs slightly. If your back needs more support, tuck a rolled hand towel beneath the center of your back.

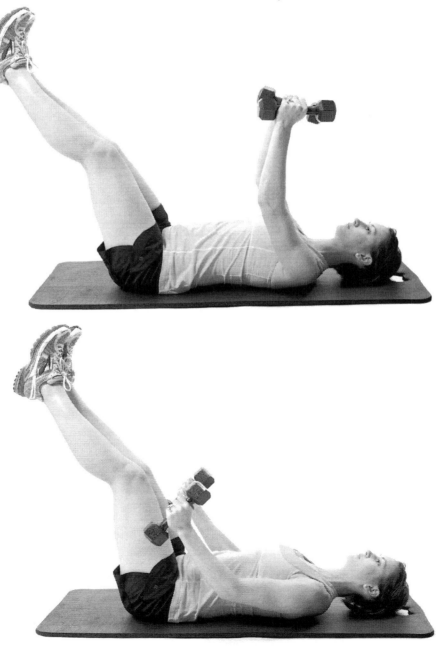

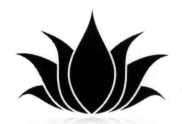

Partner Exercises

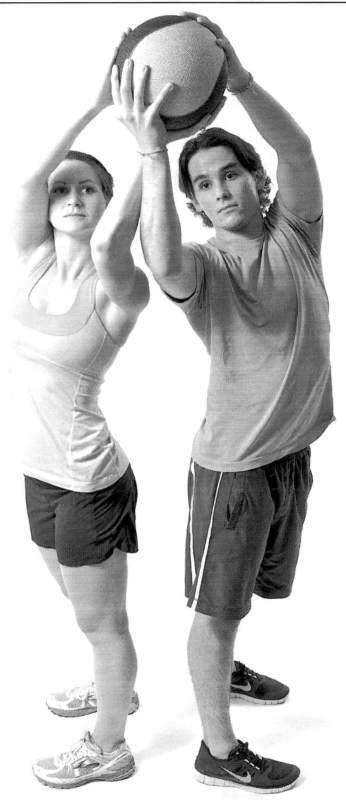

Running with a buddy is a great way to experience the road or trail. Exercising with a buddy can be just as fun. The lower-body and upper-body exercise circuits (pages 41–79) can be performed alone or with a workout partner.

The following nine exercises are designed for partners. You and a buddy can do all 10 exercises as a circuit or select a few to add to the circuits on pages 41–79.

If you're a novice, complete eight to 10 repetitions. Intermediate-level athletes should complete 10 to 12 repetitions. At the advanced level, complete 12 to 15 repetitions.

Partner Exercises

Crunch-and-Pass

Target Muscles: Rectus Abdominis, Transverse Abdominis, Lats, Hip Flexors

Place two mats end to end on the floor. You and your partner lie on the mat with heads at opposite ends and feet interlocked. Place a medicine ball on the floor above your head. This is the starting position (1). With your feet interlocked with your partner's feet, engage your core and crunch forward, bringing the ball over your head (2). Your partner crunches forward at the same time. Pass the ball to your partner before you return to the floor. Your partner takes the ball and pulls it over her head as she lies back on the floor. That's one rep. Continue passing the ball with each crunch for the desired number of reps.

Novice: 8–10 reps.

Intermediate: 10–12 reps.

Advanced: 12–15 reps.

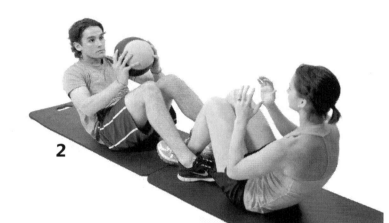

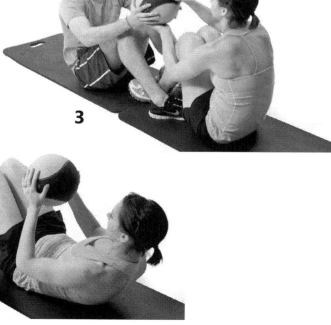

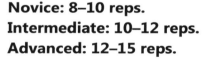

Partner Exercises

Wheelbarrow Cone Touch

Target Muscles: Core and Upper Body

Place a cone on the floor. Position yourself on your hands and knees in front of the cone. When you're ready, direct your partner to grasp both feet and lift them off the floor. Keeping your core engaged, reach out with your left hand and touch the cone, then return your hand to the floor. Next, reach out with your right hand and touch the cone. Continue touching the cone with alternating hands for 30 seconds.

Novice: 8–10 reps.

Intermediate: 10–12 reps.

Advanced: 12–15 reps.

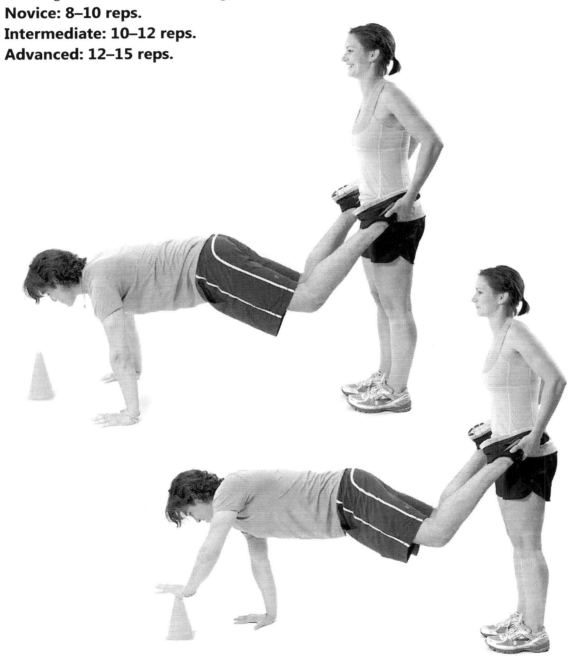

Partner Exercises

Partner Russian Twist

Target Muscles: Rectus Abdominis, Internal and External Obliques, Hip Flexors

Position two mats side by side with about a foot of space between them. Grasp a medicine ball. You and your partner each sit on a mat with knees bent and feet on the floor. Engage your core, lift your feet, and lean back 45 degrees. This is the starting position.

Looking straight ahead, move the ball as far as you can to the right (1), then swing it back across your torso toward the left, passing the ball to your partner (2), who will swing the ball as far as she can to her left (3) before swinging the ball back to her right, passing it back to you.

Continue this back-and-forth motion for 30 seconds.

Novice: 8–10 reps.
Intermediate: 10–12 reps.
Advanced: 12–15 reps.

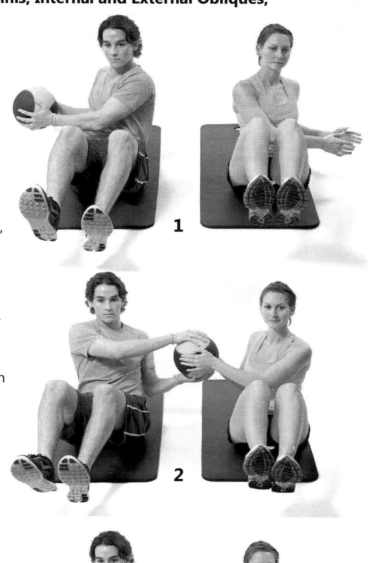

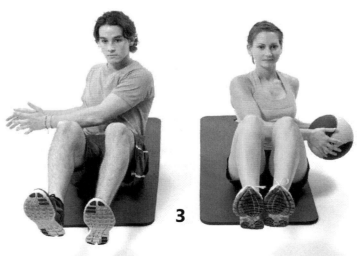

Partner Exercises

Reverse Crunch Kick-Up
Target Muscles: Rectus Abdominis; Hip Flexors; Internal and External Obliques

Lie back on the floor. Your partner stands with her feet a few inches from your ears, arms extended out and down at about a 45-degree angle and palms parallel to the floor. Grasp your partner's ankles as anchors. This is the starting position (1).

Engage your core, hold your partner's ankles, and lift both legs off the floor (keeping the knees locked). As you lift your legs, rotate them toward your partner's right hand (2). Touch your partner's hand with your feet, then lower your legs back to the floor. Repeat, aiming for your partner's left hand (3).

Alternate lifting your legs and touching your partner's hands for 30 seconds.
Novice: 8–10 reps. Intermediate: 10–12 reps. Advanced: 12–15 reps.

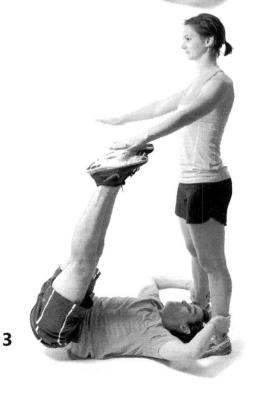

1

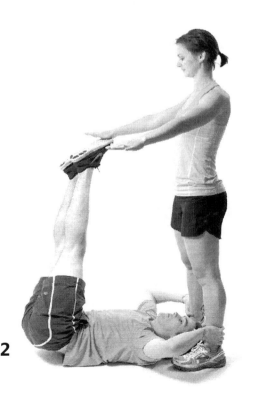

2

3

Partner Exercises

Medicine Ball High-Low Pass-Around

Target Muscles: Internal and External Obliques, Rectus Abdominis, Lats, Legs

Stand back-to-back with your partner, leaving a few inches of space in between. Pass a medicine ball to your partner over your right shoulder (1). Bend your knees and rotate your torso down to the left as your partner bends her knees and rotates her torso down and to her right (2). Reach low (about knee height) and retrieve the ball from your partner, who is also reaching low. Continue this high/low pattern for 15 seconds. Reverse the pattern by having your partner pass the ball to you over her left shoulder. Continue the reversed pattern for 15 seconds.

Novice: 8–10 reps. Intermediate: 10–12 reps. Advanced: 12–15 reps.

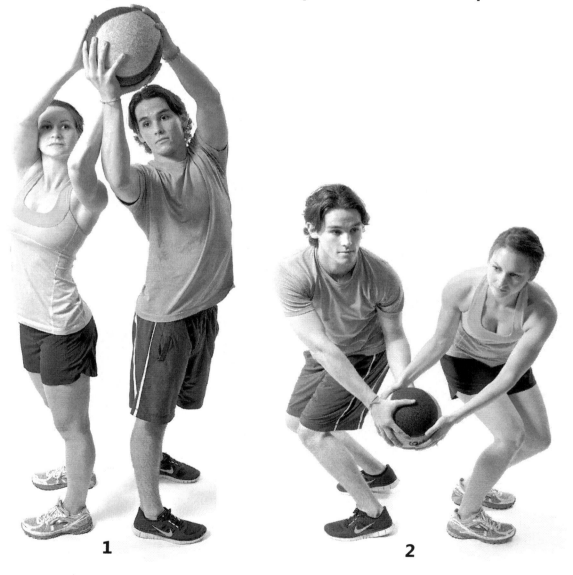

1

2

View from Opposite Side

Partner Exercises

Medicine Ball Target Crunch
Target Muscles: Internal and External Obliques, Rectus Abdominis

Grasp a small yoga or medicine ball (small enough that you can hold it with one hand). Lie back on the floor with knees bent and feet on the floor. Have your partner stand in front of you with his feet on your feet. This is the starting position (1).

Holding the ball in your left hand, crunch forward, aiming the ball toward your partner's outstretched hand (2). After touching his hand with the ball, lower your torso to the floor. That's one rep.

Continue crunching forward, aiming for your partner's hand as he changes the position with each crunch (3). Do half of the repetitions reaching with your left hand, then do the remaining half reaching with your right hand.

Novice: 8–10 reps.
Intermediate: 10–12 reps.
Advanced: 12–15 reps.

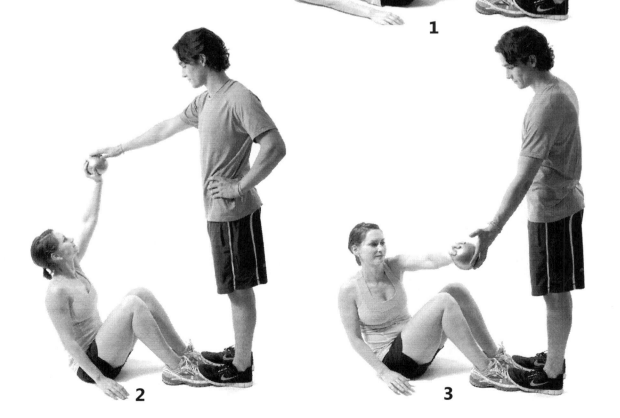

1

2

3

Partner Exercises

Partner Medicine Ball Toss

Target Muscles: Internal and External Obliques, Rectus Abdominis, Legs

Stand on a balance disk with your knees slightly bent. Your partner holds a medicine ball and stands four to five feet from your left side (1). When you're ready, have your partner toss the ball to you (2). As you catch the ball, follow its momentum and rotate your torso to the right (3). Use your obliques to pull your torso back around to the left and toss the ball back to your partner (4). That's one rep. Do half of the reps with your partner tossing the ball to your left side and half with her tossing the ball to your right side.

Novice: 8–10 reps. Intermediate: 10–12 reps. Advanced: 12–15 reps.

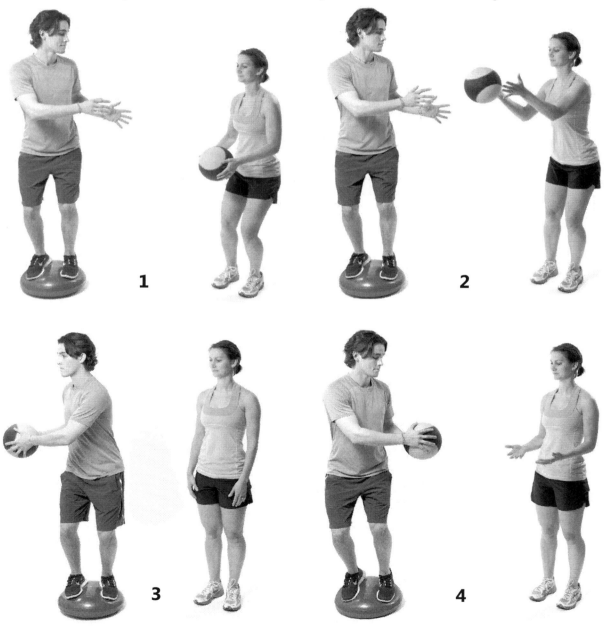

Partner Exercises

Partner Help-Up

Target Muscles: Full Body

Face your partner. Your feet should be shoulder-width apart. Grasp your partner's left hand with your left hand. Still holding hands, sit on the floor (while your partner remains standing) and roll back so that you're lying on the floor. Fully extend your left leg so that it's flat on the floor. Keep the right leg bent at the knee and the right foot planted on the floor. This is the starting position.

Without using your right hand, roll forward, driving your right foot into the floor to help you come to a standing position. (Your partner is more of a support and should not pull you up.) That's one rep. Do the desired number of reps on the right leg, then switch hands with your partner and pull up on your left leg. Then let your partner have a turn.

Novice: 8–10 reps. Intermediate: 10–12 reps. Advanced: 12–15 reps.

If using one leg is too hard, first try using both legs and work your way to using just one leg.

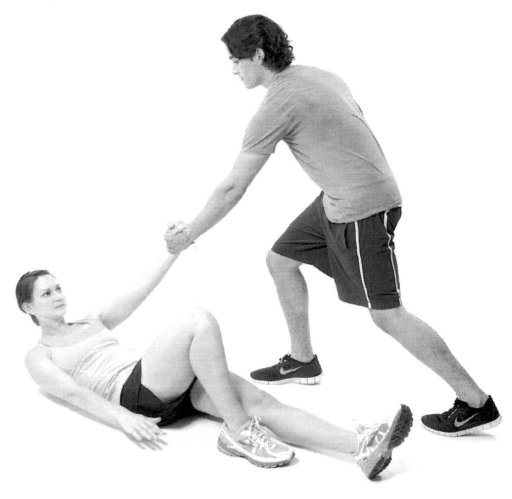

Partner Exercises

Medicine Ball Round-and-Round
Target Muscles: Rectus Abdominis, Shoulders, Lats, Legs

Lie back on the floor with your knees bent and feet off the floor. Grasp a medicine ball with both hands behind your head. Have your partner place a second medicine ball on your shins just above your ankles. This is the starting position.

Crunch forward, pulling the ball up and over your head and keeping the other ball still and positioned on your shins. Pass the ball that's in your hands to your partner (1). Next, grasp the ball from your shins and, using a controlled movement, lie back on the floor, returning the ball over your head to the floor behind you (2). While you return to the floor with the second ball, your partner places the first ball on your shins (3). That's one repetition.

Continue this cycle of crunching forward with one ball and passing it to your partner, and then taking the other ball from your shins and lying back on the floor for 30 seconds or the desired number of repetitions.
Novice: 8–10 reps. Intermediate: 10–12 reps. Advanced: 12–15 reps.

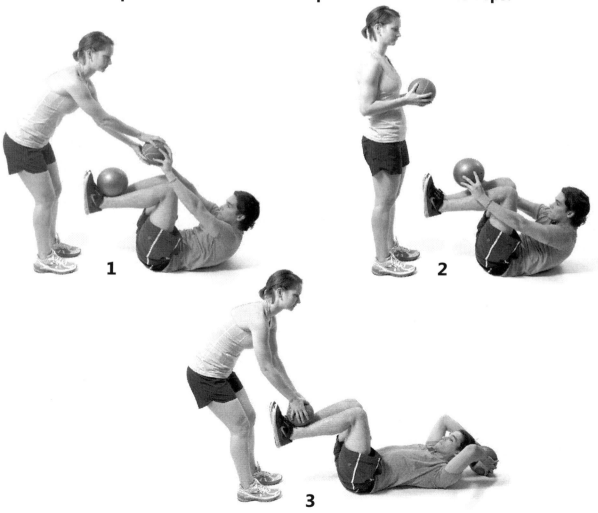

How to Fit It All In

The first question most people ask after seeing all the exercises is, "How do I fit them in?" Great question. With work, family, social events, and other commitments, it can be hard to find time for fitness.

My first response is, "You *have* to make time." Fitness needs to be the top priority. If you're not in good physical condition, then you won't be able to perform your other duties and obligations to your best ability.

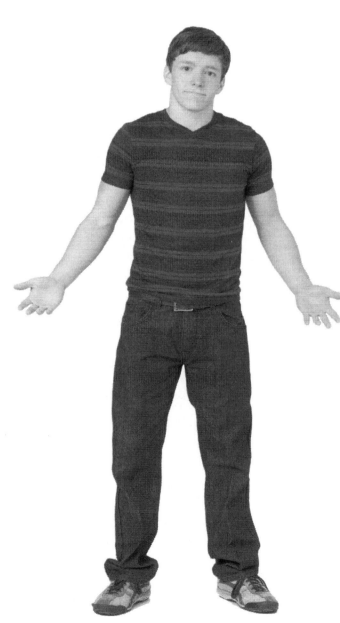

Fitness is often viewed as frivolous because of all the attention the media gives to the "perfect" body. The goal of true fitness, however, isn't cosmetic. Having a good-looking body is a nice by-product, but it's not the goal. A healthy body is the goal. Quality of life is the goal. A body that's fit for the long haul is the goal.

Good nutrition and a physically fit body work together to promote a strong immune system. A strong immune system will better defend you from illness. If you do become sick, a strong immune system will help you recover more quickly. Therefore, making time for fitness is of vital importance.

My second response is, "It takes less time than you think." You don't need hours in the gym to become physically fit. Access to a gym is great because of the availability of equipment, but you can get a great workout with a modest supply of inexpensive equipment to use at home (see pages 22–23).

The U.S. Department of Health and Human Services' *Physical Activity Guidelines for Americans* states that adults should get the following amounts of physical activity:

- Two and a half hours of **moderate-intensity aerobic activity**—working hard enough to break a sweat, or a conversational running pace.
- **Muscle-strengthening activities** that work all the major muscle groups two or more days per week.

Or

- Seventy-five minutes of **vigorous-intensity aerobic activity**. This intensity level is more demanding; conversing would be difficult.
- **Muscle-strengthening activities** that work all the major muscle groups two or more days per week.

Or

- An **equivalent mix of moderate- and vigorous-intensity aerobic activity**.
- **Muscle-strengthening activities** that work all the major muscle groups two or more days per week.

Consistency is the key to making fitness a part of your daily routine. It might take a while to find what works for you, but through trial and error, you'll find a plan of attack that fits your busy schedule.

Most weekday workouts don't need to be more than 45 minutes, so lunch can be a great time to fit them in. If midday isn't good, try early morning or on your way home from work. Many employers today encourage activities that support health and well-being. Discuss your plan to add fitness to your day with your boss or HR director. They might allow a slightly longer lunch if you make up time elsewhere during the day. Discussions like this could even lead to a fitness policy or program at your place of work, if yours doesn't already have one.

The *Physical Activity Guidelines for Americans* are a minimum recommendation. The charts on page 109 are sample maintenance plans I recommend for healthy novice, intermediate, and advanced runners who want to maintain a good running base and fit in strength training.

As you see in the sample plans, the most time required for an entire week is 4.75 hours. Compare that to other activities that eat up your available time. List your nonessential activities and nix the ones that are lowest priority. Better yet, combine them. For example, if you just can't miss that favorite TV program, then don't—but do your circuit workout while you're enjoying the show. Kids have soccer practice? No problem. Run around the soccer field while you're waiting. Be creative and I bet you'll find the time you need for your new fitness regimen.

Sample Running/Fitness Plans

Novice: Running/Fitness Plan
(3.5 hours of weekly running/fitness)

Mon	Tues	Wed	Thurs	Fri	Sat	Sun	Total Hours
Lower Body/Core Circuit 30 mins	Moderate Run 40 mins	Aerobic Cross-Training 30 mins	Moderate Run 40 mins	Upper Body/Core Circuit 30 mins	Moderate Run 40 mins	REST	2.5 hrs (Aerobic) 1 hr (Strength)

Intermediate: Running/Fitness Plan
(4 hours of weekly running/fitness)

Mon	Tues	Wed	Thurs	Fri	Sat	Sun	Total Hours
Lower Body/Core Circuit 30 mins	Moderate Run 45 mins	Aerobic Cross-Training 30 mins	Vigorous Run 45 mins	Upper Body/Core Circuit 30 mins	Long Run 60 mins	REST	3 hrs (Aerobic) 1 hr (Strength)

Advanced: Running/Fitness Plan
(4.75 hours of weekly running/fitness)

Mon	Tues	Wed	Thurs	Fri	Sat	Sun	Total Hours
Moderate Run 45 mins	Lower Body/Core Circuit 30 mins	Vigorous Run 45 mins	Aerobic Cross-Training 30 mins	Moderate Run 45 mins	Upper Body/Core Circuit 30 mins	Long Run 60+ mins	3.75+ hrs (Aerobic) 1 hr (Strength)

Moderate Run: This run gets your heart rate up to 70 percent of your maximum heart rate. It's a conversational pace, or what I like to call an "in your groove" pace.

Vigorous Run: This run gets your heart rate up to 80 to 90 percent of your maximum heart rate. A vigorous run can be as simple as adding several short bursts of speed (fartleks) to your run, or it can be a more formal workout, such as a tempo run. Other intense workouts include track intervals and hill repeats. Always begin a vigorous run with an easy 10-to-15-minute warm-up run and some dynamic stretches.

Long Run: This run builds endurance and is a little slower than a moderate run—about 65 percent of your maximum heart rate.

Aerobic Cross-Training: Any aerobic activity that's not running (for example, fitness walking, swimming, cycling, rowing, elliptical, etc.).

These plans are simply suggestions. Organize the runs to fit your schedule. A good rule of thumb, however, is never to follow a hard run or workout with another hard run or workout. Always alternate hard days with easy days.

Good Running Form

Proper running form is as important as full-body muscular endurance. They work together to help runners avoid impact-related injuries and to improve running efficiency.

When running, think of your torso or core as your center. The more you can keep your appendages (head, arms, legs, feet) near your core or center of mass, the less stress you'll put on your body while running. Less stress means less caloric expenditure (wasted energy), which means more fuel for your running.

Poor running form creates a domino effect. If your upper body is weak and has little muscular endurance, your shoulders and upper back will fatigue not far into a long run, causing you to slouch and move your head forward away from the torso. Your head weighs about eight pounds—relative to a small bowling ball. Imagine running with a bowling ball out in front of you. A similar thing happens when you round the shoulders and drop your head forward: Your head's weight pulls on your upper back, which in turn fatigues the muscles all down your back.

If your core isn't strong, then it too will fatigue with the added stress created by your slumped upper body. Once your core fatigues, your legs are left to carry all that upper-body "dead weight" and will quickly fatigue.

Ever see a runner at the end of a marathon hunched over, looking down, zombie-faced? He's probably a victim of the domino effect.

Building full-body muscular endurance, particularly in the core and upper body, and following these good running-form tips will help protect you from the domino effect.

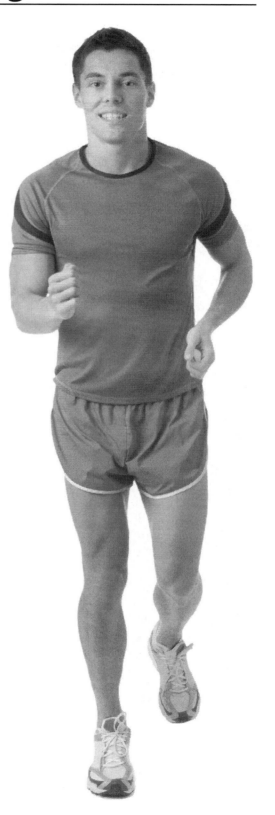

Shoulders

Strive for a tall spine, but keep the shoulders relaxed and low. Tight shoulders waste energy.

Head

Look out and down about 20 to 30 feet ahead. Avoid looking down at your feet.

Torso

Keep a tall spine for maximum lung capacity. Keep the core engaged and the shoulders back to prevent bending at the waist. If you add any lean to your stride, it should be from the ankle.

Hands

Keep hands relaxed. Cupped hands are fine, but avoid a tight fist.

Arms

Keep arms bent at 90 degrees and swinging alongside your torso. Avoid crossing your arms in front of your torso. Kick the elbows back rather than swinging your hands way out in front of your chest.

Heel Kick

Kick your heels up behind you. Think of your leg as a pendulum swinging up behind you and then down to the ground under your center of mass.

Stride

Strive for a quick turnover rather than lengthening your stride. Shoot for a cadence of 180 steps per minute.

Foot Landing

Strive for a midfoot landing that's underneath your center of mass. This allows your body to work like a shock absorber. It also allows you to immediately push off instead of having to pull forward and then push off.

Jeff Galloway's Nutrition Tips

Before, During, and After Workouts/Races

BEFORE

FUEL: Most of my run-walk clients don't need to eat anything before a morning run. In the afternoon, however, they may find their blood sugar level low and a snack beneficial. Before a run, particularly if your blood sugar level is too low, or before a race, two patterns have worked well for my athletes:

1. Within 30 minutes before exercise, eat a snack with about 100 calories of simple, easy-to-digest carbohydrates.
2. About one to two hours before a workout, have a snack that contains 150 to 250 calories. Energy bars and some fruit leather–type snacks work well.

FLUIDS: Hydrate, but don't drink too much. I recommend drinking six to eight ounces of water or coffee 90 to 120 minutes before the start of the workout, or three ounces of water within 15 minutes before the start. Drinking more than this recommended amount can lead to more pit stops during the workout or race.

PRACTICE: Don't eat or drink too much before a workout, and avoid foods that cause nausea. This will vary from runner to runner. Practice eating before long runs and faster workouts to discover what works best for you.

DURING

FUEL: Runners don't usually benefit from food or fluid during a run until the workout duration exceeds 60 minutes. During a workout exceeding 60 to 90 minutes, ingest 30 to 40 calories every 15 to 25 minutes. If you're prone to bonking (that is, low blood sugar at the end of workouts), start snacking during the first 20 minutes. Some runners may be able to wait 30 to 45 minutes before starting the boosters. Practice various eating strategies on your long runs, and pick what works best for you. A few during-the-run fuel sources are listed on the next page.

- **Gel products:** These come in small packets and are the consistency of honey or thick syrup. Because these products contain more than just sugar, some runners experience nausea when consuming them.
- **Energy bars:** Before your run, cut a bar into eight to 10 pieces. Eat a piece with a couple sips of water.
- **Candy:** Gummy bears, Life Savers, even sugar cubes are easy to digest, causing fewer nausea issues.

FLUIDS: When the run duration exceeds 90 minutes, ingest two to four ounces of water every 15 to 25 minutes. Many runners experience nausea when using sports drinks. If you have found a product that works for you, use it exactly as you have used it before.

PRACTICE: Don't eat or drink too much during a run, and avoid foods that could cause nausea. Practice eating during long runs to discover what works best for you.

AFTER

For 30 minutes after exercising, reloading circuits in the brain are turned on for maximum reloading. The quantity of calories needed is based on the duration of the workout:

- 100 calories after a 30-minute workout
- 150 calories after a 60-minute workout
- 200 calories after a two-hour workout
- 300 calories after a workout of three-plus hours

Snacks that have 80 percent simple carbohydrates and 20 percent protein are the most successful in reloading the muscles. The product that has worked best among the thousands I work with each year is Endurox R4.

For more of Jeff Galloway's information on fueling your runs, check out some of his books, such as *Running and Fat Burning for Women*; *Marathon: You Can Do It*; *Half-Marathon: You Can Do It!*; *Running Until You're 100*; and *Galloway's 5K/10K Running*.

Jeff Galloway: As a member of the 1972 Olympic team, Jeff Galloway competed against the world's best athletes in Europe, Africa, and the former Soviet Union. He broke the U.S. 10-mile record (47:49) in 1973 and has a six-mile best of 27:21. Galloway has coached more than a million runners through his books, beach retreats, running schools, Galloway training programs, and e-coaching. To receive his free e-newsletter, sign up at **JeffGalloway.com**.

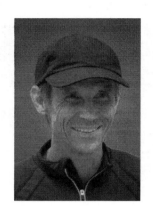

Vitamins and Minerals
Do a Runner Good

Vitamins and minerals are important to good health and play an important role in supporting an active lifestyle. While supplements can be helpful, fresh foods are the best sources of vitamins and minerals. Listed below are some of the key vitamins and minerals that runners should try to include in their daily diet.

Vitamin B6: Aids in manufacturing amino acids. Amino acids are needed to build proteins, which are essential for repairing and growing muscle tissue.
Sources: Almond butter, almonds, bananas, chicken breast, chickpeas, edamame, fortified cereals, lima beans, liver, oatmeal, peanut butter, peanuts, sunflower seeds, tomato juice, tuna, walnuts, wheat germ.

Vitamin C: Helps the immune system and aids in building and maintaining strong bones, teeth, and cartilage. Also aids in the absorption of iron.
Sources: Asparagus, beets, broccoli, carrots, cauliflower, citrus fruits, collard greens, kale, prunes, sweet potatoes, tomatoes.

Vitamin D: Aids in the absorption of vitamin C and calcium, which helps maintain healthy bone density. Also supports a strong immune system.
Sources: Almonds, almond butter, fortified milk and other dairy products, shrimp, sun exposure, wild salmon.

Vitamin E: An antioxidant that helps protect cells from oxidation damage. Vitamin C also does this, but vitamin C is water soluble whereas vitamin E is fat soluble, so together they can better help protect against cell damage. Research shows that when runners increase mileage (such as in marathon training), they need more vitamin E.
Sources: Almonds, asparagus, avocado, eggs, hazelnuts, milk, spinach, sunflower seeds, unheated vegetable oil, wheat germ, whole-grain foods.

Calcium: Vital for building strong bones in younger runners and maintaining bone density in older runners.
Sources: Almonds, arugula, avocados, broccoli, cabbage, carrots, walnuts, cashews, edamame, greens beans, kale, milk, dairy products, pumpkin, sweet potatoes, spinach.

Iron: Needed for hemoglobin production. Oxygen attaches to hemoglobin, which act like little transporters that carry oxygen from the blood to the muscles. If you're low on hemoglobin, fatigue will set in because your body isn't getting enough oxygen to the muscle where it's needed to make muscle-moving energy.

Sources: Black beans, broccoli, brown rice, chickpeas, clams, fortified cereals, green peas, kidney beans, lean cuts of red meat, lentils, oysters, pumpkin, quinoa, sardines.

Magnesium: Plays a part in building a strong immune system and strong bones; helps maintain normal muscle and nerve function; keeps heart rhythm steady; promotes normal blood pressure. It also plays a role in energy metabolism and protein synthesis.

Sources: Almonds, almond butter, artichokes, brown rice, cantaloupe, carrots, cashews, edamame, green beans, peanuts, peanut butter, walnuts, yogurt.

Omega-3 fatty acids: Omega-3s have many health benefits, but their role as an anti-inflammatory is one of the most important for runners. They also support good blood circulation.

Sources: Brussels sprouts, cabbage, cauliflower, cod, cooked soybeans, dried ground cloves, dried ground oregano, flaxseed oil, flaxseed, halibut, mustard seeds, salmon, walnuts.

Potassium: Works with sodium to maintain the body's water and electrolyte balance. A potassium deficiency can contribute to dehydration, which can cause fatigue, lack of energy, and muscle cramping.

Sources: Apples, apricots, artichokes, bananas, beets, cashews, chickpeas, coconut water (100 percent only), edamame, eggplant, figs, grapes, green beans, guava, honeydew melon, oatmeal, pumpkin.

The Protein Myth

Protein is easily one of the most overused supplements. Supplement advertisements have the public believing that protein makes muscle bigger. This is very misleading. Protein doesn't zoom to your muscles and magically make them grow bigger. Protein does, however, help rebuild and repair muscle fibers. After a hard workout, protein is a necessary ingredient in the muscle-rebuilding process, which makes muscles stronger. Protein is found in muscles, bone, blood, hormones, antibodies, and enzymes. Protein also helps regulate the body's water balance and transport nutrients, supports brain function, and makes muscles contract. Protein also helps keep the body healthy by fighting off disease. Important for runners, protein helps produce stamina and energy, which can keep fatigue at bay.

Protein is definitely a key ingredient for a strong, healthy body, especially if you're in training. Research has shown, however, that the body has a limit at which it stops using extra protein. Studies have found that the body maxes out at two grams of protein per kilogram of body weight. If you take more than that, your body voids it, unused, as waste. Only individuals such as bodybuilders doing heavy resistance training need that higher level of two grams per kilogram of body weight. Endurance runners need protein in the range of .8 to 1.5 grams per kilogram of body weight. Sedentary people need only .8 grams per kilogram of body weight.

An average male runner who weighs 175 pounds needs 64 to 119 grams of protein per day. That might still seem like a lot of protein to ingest during a day, but remember that one cup of tuna has almost 40 grams of protein. A cup of black bean soup contains about 12 grams of protein. It doesn't take long to get enough protein just by eating a healthy diet. Vegetarians may have to be a little more diligent in making sure they get the required daily amount of protein.

If you're eating a well-balanced diet with a variety of fruits, vegetables, lean meats, whole grains, and healthy fats, then you're probably getting everything that big canister of powdered protein has to offer. So why not go the natural route?

Carbohydrates Are Your Friend

For a while now, carbohydrates have gotten a bad rap. The rising popularity of low- and no-carb diets has given the general public the impression that carbs are their enemy. Carbs are like anything: In excess they can be bad.

Your body needs carbohydrates to function properly. Carbs provide fuel for the body. They also help regulate the metabolism of protein and fat. If the body does not receive sufficient carbohydrates, it could begin breaking down protein for energy production. Protein can be used as fuel, but it's not very efficient, and when protein is used as fuel, less is available for its main function—rebuilding and repair. The protein-sparing action of carbohydrates protects the body's stores of protein.

More important, command central—your brain—needs carbohydrates for proper function. Through the digestion process, carbohydrates are converted to glucose. Glucose is the fuel on which the body functions. Unlike other muscles in the body, the brain can't store glucose. Instead, it depends on a steady supply of glucose from the blood circulating through the body. Ever feel light-headed during an afternoon workout and then realize you skipped lunch? That light-headed feeling might be the result of low blood sugar, which means you're low on that steady supply of glucose in the blood flowing to the brain. Not a good feeling. When you eat something, that light-headedness usually subsides.

There are "good carbs" and "bad carbs." It's the bad (simple) carbs that give the good (complex) carbs a bad rap. Unfortunately, simple carbs are prevalent in our diet. They are found in convenience foods such as cakes, cookies, crackers, breads, and so on. Foods such these are made with refined/processed grains, which are quickly digested and converted to fat in the body unless activity ensues soon after ingestion.

Complex carbs take longer to digest; therefore, the body has more time to use them as fuel. These include vegetables and whole grains. Complex carbs are also high in fiber, which has many benefits for the body.

Forty-five to 65 percent of your daily calories should come from carbohydrates. That's about 225 to 325 grams of carbs per day. The USDA recommends a minimum of 130 grams of carbohydrates per day. To get a better idea of how that correlates to portion sizes, MyPlate.gov recommends that adults eat 2.5 cups of vegetables, two cups of fruit, and six ounces of grains every day. When working out intensely or training for a race, your carb intake should be closer to 65 percent. On days when you're not working out or running, your carb intake should be closer to 45 percent.

When shopping for complex carbohydrate products such as bread or pasta, look for 100 percent whole grain or 100 percent whole wheat. If it's unclear how much whole grain a food contains, check the nutrition label. Low fiber means more refined (or processed) grains. Also check to make sure the sugar content is low. Then check the ingredients list. The ingredients are listed in order of how much the product contains. "Whole grain" or "whole wheat" should be listed as the first ingredient. If you're still not sure, buy products that have the highest fiber content per serving (at least three grams or more).

Products that contain 100 percent whole wheat will also contain more protein since the grains have not been refined. Try to find products offering at least eight grams of protein. Whole-grain foods also provide many important vitamins and minerals, such as vitamin E, iron, magnesium, potassium, and phosphorus, just to name a few.

Avoid products made of "enriched flour" or "enriched bleached flour." That means refined grains have been used. These grains have been stripped of most of their fiber, vitamins, and minerals. "Enriched" sounds good, but it really means that some of the vitamins and minerals have been added back to the flour. Fiber, however, can't be added back to the flour.

As previously mentioned, raw or cooked vegetables are great sources of complex carbohydrates. Technically, fruits are a simple carbohydrate, but that doesn't mean they are bad. Whole fruit is full of fiber and is nutrient dense, so while the body may digest it more quickly, whole fruit is a great source of both carbohydrates and fiber. Go light on fruit juice. Even if it's 100 percent fruit juice, this very concentrated version of the fruit greatly increases the sugar content. Whole fruit (fresh or frozen) is a better choice. Dried fruits are also a great choice. Dairy products such as skim milk and cheese are more good sources of carbohydrates.

Find more ideas for complex carbohydrates to add to your diet on pages 122–124.

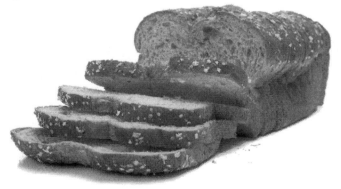

"Wise Choice" Foods for Runners

Keeping the cupboard and fridge stocked with healthy choices is a great way to ensure proper eating at home. If you're like most people, if a food is in the pantry or fridge, you'll eventually eat it, no matter what it is. But if your kitchen is stocked with healthy options, you can't go wrong.

Shopping can become routine, just like the rest of our lives. We can get into a rut with our food choices. The following pages include suggestions for "wise-choice" foods from all the food categories that runners—and everyone, for that matter—can stock up on. These aren't the only foods that are good to have on hand, but they're a great start.

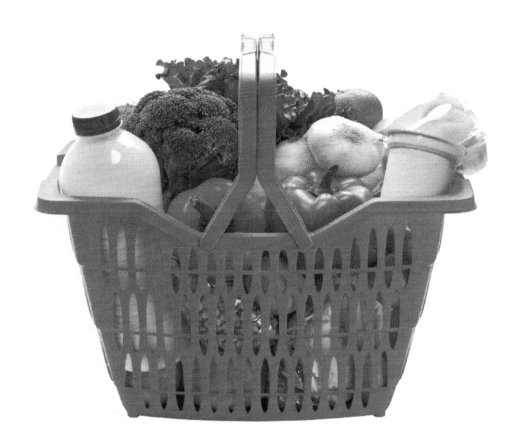

FRUIT

Fruit is a great source of simple carbs. Yep, that's right, simple carbs. Simple carbs usually conjure images of white bread and doughnuts. Fruit contains fructose, which is a simple sugar, but unlike a doughnut, fruit is nutrient dense and packed with fiber and antioxidants. Fresh fruit is best, but frozen is a close second. Dried fruit is also an excellent choice.

Fruit makes a great fuel source just before or after a workout. Its simple sugar is quickly digested and converted to energy needed for your workout or for rebuilding after your workout.

Along with nuts and seeds, fruit makes a delicious addition to any salad, cup of yogurt, or hot cereal. Fruit is perfect in smoothies and makes a healthy sweet dessert. Listed below are the fruits you should include on your shopping list.

- **Apples** (vitamin C, antioxidants)
- **Apricots** (vitamins A and C, potassium)
- **Avocados** (vitamin A, potassium, folate)
- **Bananas** (vitamins C and B6, potassium, manganese)
- **Black olives** (anti-inflammatory; improves immune function)
- **Blueberries, blackberries, and raspberries** (vitamins C and K, calcium, magnesium, potassium, and anthocyanin, which works as an anti-inflammatory and may help protect against Alzheimer's disease)
- **Cantaloupe** (vitamins A, B1, B3, B6, C, and K; potassium; magnesium; folate)
- **Cherries** (vitamin C, potassium)
- **100% coconut water** (potassium, sodium, magnesium, calcium, phosphorus)
- **Figs** (vitamin B6, iron, calcium, potassium, manganese)
- **Grapes** (vitamins C, A, and K; potassium; magnesium; calcium,)
- **Oranges** (vitamins A, B1, and C; potassium; calcium)
- **Peaches** (vitamins A, C, and K; potassium; calcium; magnesium; beta-carotene)
- **Pineapple** (vitamins B1, B6, and C; magnesium)
- **Prunes** (vitamins A and C, potassium, iron)
- **Raisins** (potassium, fiber, protein)

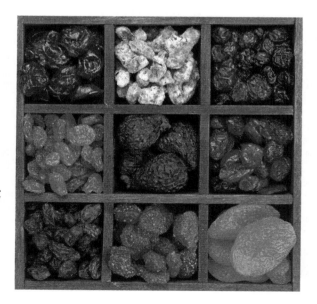

VEGETABLES

Vegetables are an excellent source of complex carbohydrates, fiber, and other nutrients. Listed below are just a few options to keep in your kitchen. Fresh is best, but frozen is also a good choice. Canned veggies such as kidney, black, and pinto beans are perfect for quick and healthy soups, stews, and chili.

- **Asparagus** (vitamins C and K, folic acid)
- **Kidney beans** (protein, potassium, iron)
- **Black beans** (protein, potassium, iron)
- **Pinto beans** (protein, potassium, iron)
- **Garbanzo beans, aka chickpeas** (protein, potassium, iron)
- **Edamame** (protein, potassium, iron)
- **Lentils** (protein, folate, very high in fiber)
- **Bell peppers** (vitamins A, B6, and C)
- **Broccoli** (vitamins C, K, A, and B6; potassium; riboflavin; manganese; folate)
- **Butternut squash** (vitamins A, C, and E; potassium)
- **Carrots** (vitamins A, B1, B3, B6, C, E, and K; potassium; lutein; beta-carotene)
- **Cauliflower** (vitamins B6, C, and K; folate)
- **Celery** (vitamins K and C, potassium)
- **Corn** (vitamin C, fiber, potassium)
- **Cucumber** (vitamin K)
- **Leafy greens: romaine, Swiss chard, kale, spinach, mustard greens** (vitamins A, C, and K; potassium, iron)
- **Onions** (vitamins B6 and C; chromium, which helps lower insulin levels)
- **Potatoes** (vitamins B6 and C, potassium, magnesium, manganese, niacin, folate)
- **Pumpkin** (vitamin A, potassium, beta-carotene, calcium, iron)
- **Summer squash and zucchini** (vitamins C and B6, potassium)
- **Sweet potatoes** (vitamins A and C, potassium, beta-carotene, iron)
- **Tomatoes** (vitamins A, C, and K; potassium; lycopene)

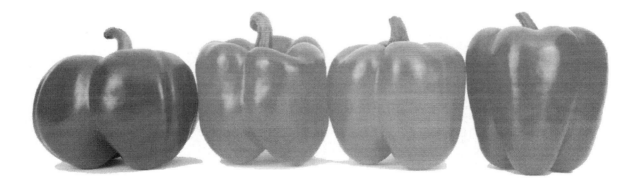

GRAINS

Look for 100 percent whole grain or 100 percent whole wheat. If it's not clear how much whole grain is used, check the nutrition label. Buy products that contain the highest fiber content per serving (three grams or more). Products containing 100 percent whole wheat also have more protein since the grains have not been refined. Try to find products with at least eight grams of protein.

Avoid products made of "enriched flour" or "enriched bleached flour," which means the product is made from refined grains. These grains have been stripped of most of their fiber, vitamins, and minerals. "Enriched" sounds good, but it really means that some of the vitamins and minerals have been added back to the flour. Fiber can't be added back to the flour.

- **100% whole-wheat pita bread**
- **100% whole-wheat, whole-grain, or whole-grain corn flour tortillas**
- **100% whole-wheat crackers**
- **100% whole-wheat bagels**
- **100% whole-wheat English muffins**
- **100% whole-wheat or whole-grain pasta**
- **Omega-3-enhanced pasta**
- **Barley**
- **Brown rice**
- **Black rice** (Loaded with vitamin E and antioxidants.)
- **Couscous**
- **Grits** (Choose stone-ground grits—they have more vitamins and minerals.)
- **Low-sugar whole-grain cereal** (Cold or hot.)
- **Pretzels** (Choose the baked whole-grain variety.)
- **Oatmeal** (Steel-cut is probably the most healthful, but the quick-cooking and instant varieties are also good. Check the fat and sodium content of instant varieties.)
- **Quinoa** (Besides soybeans, quinoa is the only other plant that's a complete protein. It cooks quickly and can be used as a replacement in many pasta and rice dishes. It can also be prepared as a tasty hot breakfast cereal.)

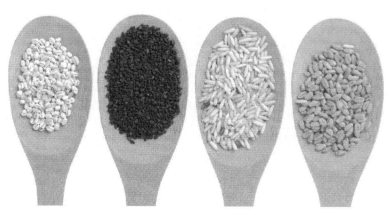

DAIRY

Dairy products are excellent sources of protein and calcium, necessary for strong bones. Calcium is also a key ingredient in the energy production process for muscle contraction. Choose low-fat or no-fat varieties. Milk is fortified with vitamin D, which helps build a strong immune system.

- **Skim milk**
- **Part-skim mozzarella string cheese**
- **1% or fat-free cottage cheese**
- **Kefir** (Best described as a liquid "drinkable" yogurt.)
- **Low-fat or fat-free traditional yogurt and Greek yogurt** (Both traditional and Greek yogurt contain healthy live bacteria that promote good digestive health and are great sources of calcium and protein. Greek yogurt contains twice the protein of traditional yogurt.)
- **Low-fat chocolate milk** (Contains the perfect four-to-one ratio of carbs to protein, making it a great post-run recovery snack.)

SEEDS, NUTS, and NUT BUTTERS

Nuts are a great source of protein, vitamin E, vitamins B1 and B6, folate, potassium, and magnesium. They also provide a small amount of fiber and iron. Nuts are a rich source of heart-healthy fats (mono- and polyunsaturated) and omega-3s, which help lower artery-clogging LDL cholesterol. Keep the serving size small—about one ounce—and eat raw or toasted varieties that contain no additional oils or salt. A great way to add nuts to your diet is to toss one ounce into a salad, your morning bowl of oatmeal or yogurt, or a pasta dish. A small square of dark chocolate and an ounce of almonds make a great snack!

- **Almonds**
- **Almond butter**
- **Cashews**
- **Chia seeds**
- **Hazelnuts**
- **Peanuts**
- **Peanut butter**
- **Pecans**
- **Pine nuts**
- **Pistachios**
- **Pumpkins seeds**
- **Sunflower seeds**
- **Walnuts**

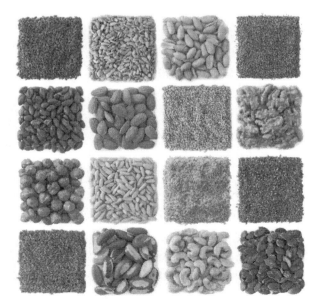

MEAT, FISH, EGGS, and MEAT SUBSTITUTES

Meat, fish, eggs, and meat substitutes are good sources of complete proteins. Fish containing omega-3s (healthy polyunsaturated fats), like salmon, tuna, and sardines, help improve cardiovascular health. Lean meats and poultry are high in iron, vitamins B6 and B12, zinc, and phosphorus. Research shows that eggs aren't the bad guys we once thought—an egg a day is fine. They're high in protein, iron, vitamin B12, and folate, and are rich in vitamin K, which promotes good bone health.

- **Fresh or frozen chicken or turkey breast** (Contains selenium, which helps protect muscles from cell damage caused by free radicals.)
- **Rotisserie chicken breast**
- **Lean cuts of red meat** (Rich in iron.)
- **Deli-sliced turkey, ham, roast beef** (Watch sodium and fat levels.)
- **Ground turkey or chicken** (Select brands made of lean white meat.)
- **Salmon, tuna, halibut, sardines** (Good sources of omega-3s and vitamin D. Select varieties packed in water.)
- **Veggie patties**
- **Eggs and egg substitutes** (Egg yolk contains the fat, including omega-3s, as well as vitamins A, B12, and E, and about three-fourths of the egg's calories. The white contains more than half of the protein, iron, and selenium. Eggs also contain choline, which may help reduce inflammation.)

SPICES and SEASONINGS

- **Cilantro** (vitamin K)
- **Cumin** (calcium, iron, magnesium)
- **Curry powder** (A spice blend including cayenne or red pepper, coriander, cumin, and turmeric.)
- **Garlic** (Helps lower LDL cholesterol.)
- **Ginger** (Anti-inflammatory; relieves gastrointestinal distress.)
- **Oregano** (vitamin K, fiber, iron, and calcium)
- **Rosemary** (Anti-inflammatory.)
- **Thyme** (Antioxidants; protects against cell damage and inflammation.)
- **Turmeric** (Anti-inflammatory; contains iron and manganese.)

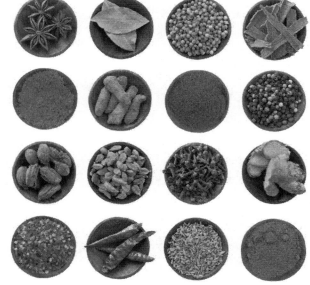

MORE HEALTHY FOODS

- **Blackstrap molasses:** This by-product of the sugar-making process is low in sugar and loaded with nutrients like iron, potassium, calcium, and magnesium.
- **Honey:** A natural alternative sweetener; raw, unfiltered honey is best.
- **Dark chocolate:** Contains heart-healthy flavonols. Choose varieties made of 70 percent or more cocoa. Keep the serving size small.
- **Energy bars:** Convenient energy source. Select bars with six grams or less of fat, at most 200 calories, 25 to 30 grams of carbs, and five to 10 grams of protein.
- **Extra virgin olive oil:** Helps to lower LDL and raise HDL cholesterol.
- **Guacamole:** A good source of potassium, vitamin E, heart-healthy unsaturated fats, and folate.
- **Hummus:** Made with chickpeas and tahini (sesame paste), hummus is a great source of protein and calcium.
- **Popcorn:** Make your own air-popped corn.
- **Salsa:** Choose the freshly made varieties found in the refrigerated produce section.
- **Sports drinks:** Good for fueling up before and during a run and for refueling after run. If you're using a sports drink for fuel, be sure to select varieties that are not low in carbs.
- **Tomato-based pasta sauce:** Potassium; vitamins A, C, and K; and antioxidants. Meat sauces also provide some protein. Select sauces with fewer than 700 milligrams of sodium per half cup.
- **Trail mix:** Swap varieties that include candy for mixes consisting of dried fruit, granola, seeds, and nuts.

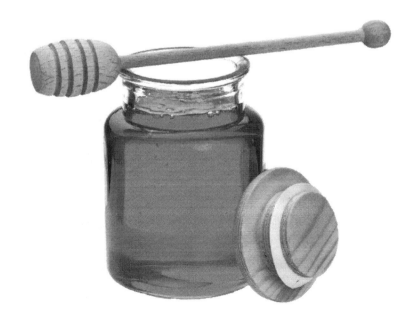

Snack Ideas for Before, During, and After Running

Eating properly to fuel your runs is vital, especially for longer runs. Every runner has different taste, smell, and texture preferences as well as food sensitivities. There is no single "right" food to eat while running.

The best method is to learn by trial and error. If you're preparing for a race, use the training period to test out various foods before, during, and after your run. Never try anything new on race day.

The following pages provide healthy food ideas for before, during, and after running. Try a few and see which work best for you.

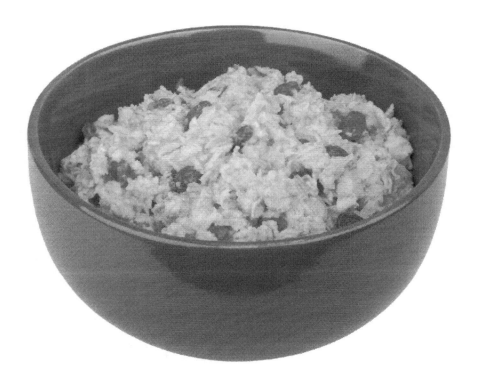

Before Your Run

90 minutes to 2 hours before running:
Eat 30 to 80 grams of carbs.

- Bagel with peanut or almond butter
- English muffin with peanut butter or almond butter and fruit preserves
- Waffle with peanut butter or almond butter
- Banana sandwich with peanut butter
- Graham crackers with peanut butter or almond butter
- Oatmeal with added nuts and fruit
- One egg on an English muffin
- Hard-boiled egg and toast with preserves
- Dry cereal and fruit (Add milk if dairy doesn't bother you on the run.)
- Energy bar with sports drink
- Greek or traditional yogurt with fruit and/or granola
- Small container of yogurt and a banana slathered with peanut butter
- Yogurt fruit smoothie

30 to 60 minutes before running:
Eat foods that are quickly and easily digested.

- Animal crackers or Teddy Grahams with water or sports drink
- Sports drink
- Energy bar (Eat bars that are low in fat/protein soon before running.)
- Energy gel
- Fruit (A medium orange is great; choose whole fruit over juice.)
- Small container of traditional yogurt with fruit and/or granola
- Handful of pretzels
- Peanut butter crackers (two or three)
- Fig bar

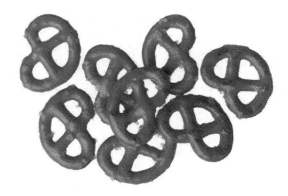

During Your Run

Keep energy stores topped off during long runs with the following:

- Energy gels
- Sports drink
- Gummy bears or jelly beans
- Tootsie Rolls
- Pretzels
- Energy bars (low-fat, low-protein varieties)
- Fig bars
- Gingersnaps
- Rice Krispie treats
- Bagel

After Your Run

Refueling within 30 minutes after running is vital for providing your body with the energy required to begin rebuilding. Select foods that provide a four-to-one ratio of carbs to protein (about 40 to 80 grams of carbs and 10 to 20 grams of protein).

- Eight ounces skim or low-fat chocolate milk
- Peanut butter and jelly sandwich and skim milk
- Bagel with peanut butter, almond butter, or Nutella
- Whole-wheat crackers and peanut or almond butter
- Brown rice pudding and a banana
- Bowl of cereal and milk
- Turkey sandwich
- Hard-boiled egg, toast, and fruit or juice
- Peanut butter and banana sandwich
- Fruit and yogurt smoothie
- Fruit smoothie with protein powder
- Energy bar and sports drink
- Trail mix

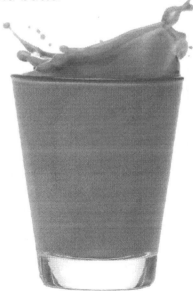

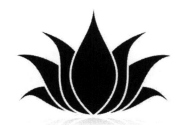

Recipes from the Experts

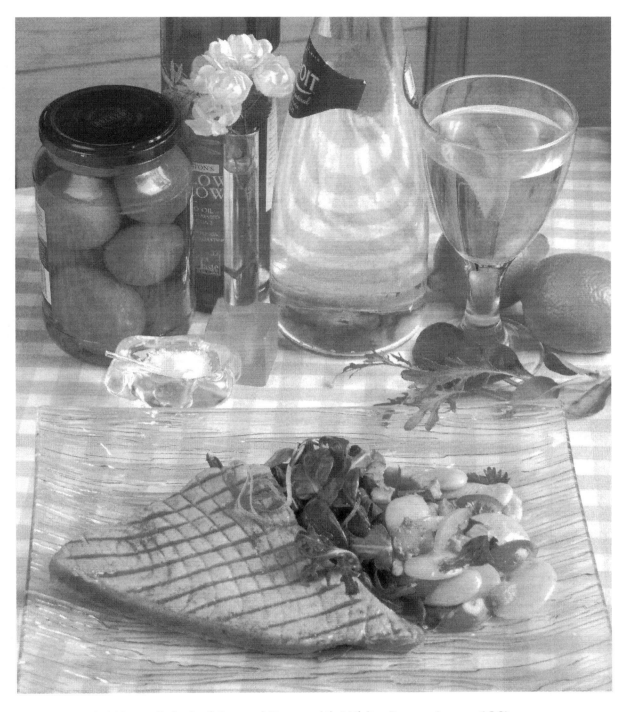

Kate Percy's Warm Salad of Seared Tuna with White Beans (page 138)
Photo courtesy of Kate Percy

Dean Karnazes's Monkey Flip Recovery Smoothie

Packed with electrolytes, protein, and carbs, this mild-tasting smoothie is delicious without being overpowering. It's one of my favorite recovery beverages. I recommend using ZICO Natural Coconut water for the best balance of natural electrolytes and sugars.

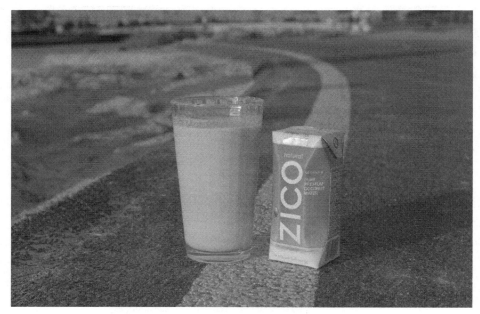

Photo courtesy of ZICO Pure Premium Coconut Water

Ingredients
11 ounces 100% coconut water
1 banana
1 tablespoon almond butter
2 teaspoons plain nonfat Greek yogurt
Stevia or honey to taste
Ice to preference

Directions
Add all ingredients to a blender. Blend until smooth.
Makes 1 serving.

Dean Karnazes: *Time* magazine named Dean Karnazes as one of the "Top 100 Most Influential People in the World." *Men's Fitness* hailed him as one of the fittest men on the planet. An internationally recognized endurance athlete and best-selling author, Dean has pushed his body and mind to inconceivable limits. Among his many accomplishments, he has run 350 continuous miles, forgoing sleep for three nights. He's run across Death Valley in 120-degree heat, and he's run a marathon to the South Pole in negative 40 degrees. On 10 different occasions, he's run a 200-mile relay race solo, racing alongside teams of 12.

His most recent endeavor was running 50 marathons in all 50 U.S. states in 50 consecutive days, finishing with the New York City Marathon, which he ran in three hours flat.

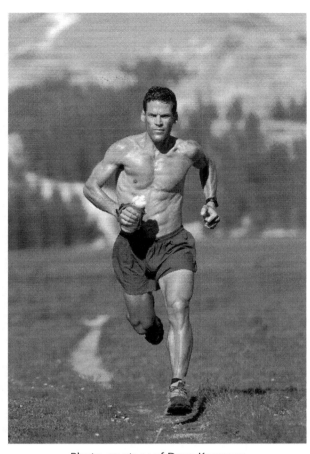

Photo courtesy of Dean Karnazes

Dean and his incredible adventures have been featured on *60 Minutes*, *Late Show with David Letterman*, *CBS News*, CNN, ESPN, the *Howard Stern Show*, NPR's *Morning Edition*, the BBC, and many others. He has appeared on the cover of *Runner's World* and *Outside*, and has been featured in *Time*, *Newsweek*, *People*, *GQ*, *New York Times*, *USA Today*, *Washington Post*, *Men's Journal*, *Forbes*, *Chicago Tribune*, *Los Angeles Times*, and *London Telegraph*, to mention a few. He is a monthly columnist for *Men's Health*, the largest men's publication in the world.

Beyond being a celebrated endurance athlete, philanthropist, and best-selling author, Dean is an accomplished businessman with a notable professional career. He has worked for Fortune 500 companies and startups alike. A graduate of University of San Francisco's McLaren School of Management, with additional graduate-level coursework at Stanford University, he is uniquely able to demonstrate how the lessons learned from athletics can be applied to business, and he is able to convey, with authenticity, the many insights he has gleaned along the way as an athlete.

Sage Rountree's Thumbprint Nut Cookies

Ingredients
1 cup unbleached flour
2 cups almonds, coarsely ground
4 cups rolled oats
1/2 teaspoon salt
1 cup maple syrup
1 cup canola oil
1/2 cup jam (I like raspberry)

Directions
1. Preheat oven to 350 degrees Fahrenheit.
2. In a medium bowl, combine flour, almonds, oats, and salt.
3. In another bowl, mix together the syrup and oil. Add to the dry ingredients and mix well. Let dough stand for 15 minutes or chill it in the refrigerator for a day or two.
4. Roll dough into 3/4-inch balls and arrange on baking sheets. Make a little dent in the top of each ball and fill with 1/2 teaspoon (or less) of the jam.
5. Bake for 15 minutes or until slightly brown. Let cookies cool before eating—hot jelly burns!

Makes approximately 5 dozen cookies. Adapted from *Tassajara Cookbook* by Karla Oliveira (Gibbs Smith, 2007).

Sage Rountree is an internationally recognized authority in yoga for athletes and an endurance sports coach specializing in athletic recovery. She is also the author of numerous books, including *The Athlete's Guide to Yoga*, and she writes for publications such as *Runner's World*, *Yoga Journal*, and *USA Triathlon Life*. Her classes, training plans, videos, books, and articles make yoga and endurance exercise accessible to everyone. Her goal is to help people find the right balance between work and rest for peak performance in sports and in life. An experienced registered yoga teacher with the Yoga Alliance, Sage is a faculty member at the Kripalu Center for Yoga and Health. Her nationwide workshops include weekends on yoga for athletes, training yoga teachers on working with athletes, and running and yoga retreats. Her students include casual athletes, Olympians, NBA and NFL players, and many University of North Carolina athletes and coaches. Sage lives with her husband and daughters in Chapel Hill, North Carolina, and co-owns the Carrboro Yoga Company and the Durham Yoga Company.

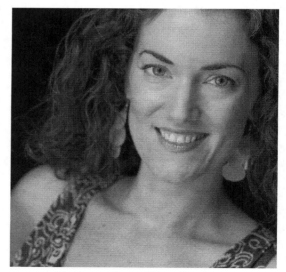

Photo courtesy of Sage Rountree

Danny Dreyer's Chi Smoothie

This is my favorite drink after a long run. I will say up front that I have a Vitamix, which is a godsend for us when making smoothie-type drinks.

Ingredients
1/2 cup frozen (or fresh) organic blueberries (antioxidant)
1/2 cup frozen (or fresh) organic strawberries (vitamin C)
1/4 cup crushed organic hemp seeds (high in protein, omega-6, omega-3)
1 heaping tablespoon organic chia seeds (high in protein, omega-3, antioxidants, polynutrients)
8 ounces pure organic pomegranate juice (antioxidant)
1/2 banana (good source of potassium)
1 teaspoon raw organic cacao (super antioxidant, high in zinc)

Directions
In a blender, combine all ingredients and blend on medium speed for 2 to 3 minutes. If using frozen fruit, you can add a little hot water to avoid brain freeze.

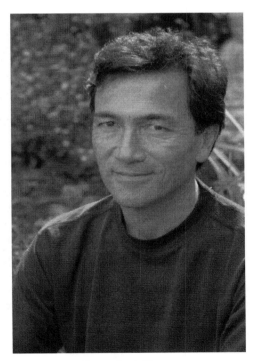

Danny Dreyer is the cofounder of ChiRunning and ChiWalking, revolutionary forms of moving that blend the subtle inner focuses of tai chi with running and walking. His work is based on his study of tai chi with Master Zhu Xilin and internationally renowned Master George Xu, and his 35 years of experience, running, racing ultramarathons, and coaching people in "intelligent movement." He has taught thousands of people the ChiRunning and ChiWalking techniques with profound results.

Danny is the author or numerous books, including *ChiRunning: A Revolutionary Approach to Effortless, Injury-Free Running*; *ChiWalking: Five Mindful Steps to Lifelong Health and Energy*; and *ChiMarathon: The Breakthrough Natural Running Program for a Pain-Free Half Marathon and Marathon*.

Photo: Lori Cheung

Kate Percy's Warm Salad of Seared Tuna with White Beans

An ideal addition to your summer training diet, this delicious and nutritious meal is balanced and packed with complex, low-GI carbohydrates, omega-3 fatty acids, vitamins, protein, fiber, and minerals such as potassium and iron. White beans are a welcome alternative to rice or pasta. They provide slow-burning carbohydrates to sustain energy levels and minerals that are vital for replacing nutrients lost through sweat during the hotter months.

Ingredients
100 grams (about 3.5 ounces or 1/2 cup) pancetta cubes
2 tablespoons olive oil, divided
2 cloves garlic, peeled and crushed
2 (15-ounce) cans butter beans
4 sun-dried tomatoes, chopped (use fresh tomatoes as an alternative)
2 tablespoons lemon juice
Large handful flat-leaf parsley, chopped
Salt and freshly ground black pepper to taste
2 tablespoons balsamic vinegar
4 tablespoons extra-virgin olive oil
2 preserved lemons, finely sliced, pulp removed, plus a little brine for the dressing
1 bunch arugula and/or spinach
4 thick tuna steaks

Directions
1. Gently saute pancetta in 1 tablespoon olive oil for 5 minutes until cooked. Add garlic, beans, tomatoes, lemon juice, and half of the parsley; heat through. Season with salt and pepper.
2. Make the dressing by mixing together the balsamic vinegar, 4 tablespoons extra-virgin olive oil, preserved lemon, the rest of the parsley, salt, pepper, and preserved lemon brine (1 to 2 teaspoons) to taste. On four plates (this recipe looks good in large flat-bottomed pasta bowls), arrange the arugula and/or spinach and spoon on the white bean mixture.
3. Lightly brush tuna with remaining 1 tablespoon olive oil. In a very hot griddle or frying pan, fry the steaks for a couple minutes on each side. Don't overcook. They should be pink inside and will continue to cook slightly after you have removed them from the pan.
4. Place a steak on top of each bed of beans and generously drizzle with the dressing.

Makes 4 servings. (See a photo of this dish on page 133.)

Kate Percy's Banana Recovery Shake

Simple but effective, this shake has an ideal carbohydrate-to-protein ratio to kick-start the recovery process after a long workout when muscle glycogen levels are depleted. It provides carbs to replenish glycogen levels and protein to repair muscle cells. It's quickly and easily digested, virtually fat-free, and packed with vitamins C and B6 and essential minerals like potassium and calcium to replace lost electrolytes.

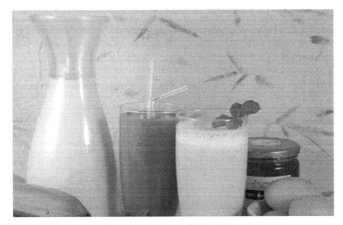

Photo courtesy of Kate Percy

Ingredients

1 egg white
1 very ripe banana, roughly chopped
2 ice cubes or 1 tablespoon crushed ice
200 milliliters (about 1 cup) skim milk
1 teaspoon honey
3 teaspoons chocolate syrup or squeeze of lime (optional)

Directions

In a blender, combine all ingredients. Blend at full speed until smooth. Pour into a chilled glass and serve.

Makes 1 serving.

Kate Percy, marathon runner, cook, and author, is passionate about the link between good eating and better athletic performance and the vital role food plays in fueling stamina and recovery. Kate's recent book, *Go Faster Food*, offers advice for endurance sports enthusiasts on how to eat for optimal training, performance, and recovery through hundreds of delicious, imaginative, and energy-boosting recipes.

Kate's recipes and ideas on eating for fitness have been published in the national press. She's also a regular contributor to *Cycling Plus, Cycling Weekly, FHM, Men's Health, Men's Fitness, Triathlon Plus, Runner's World, Running Free*, and *Health and Fitness Magazine*.

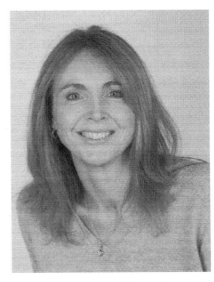

Photo courtesy of Kate Percy

Troy Busot's Turkey Chili

This hearty, easy-to-make recipe is full of veggies and lean protein and makes a great training meal.

Ingredients
1 tablespoon olive oil
1 cup chopped onions
1 cup diced red bell pepper
1 cup diced green bell pepper
1/2 cup diced carrots
1 clove garlic, finely chopped
2 tablespoons chili powder
3 teaspoons ground cumin
1 pound ground turkey breast
1 (16-ounce) container of mild salsa
3 cups reduced-sodium, fat-free chicken broth
2 (16-ounce) cans black beans, drained and rinsed, or 3 3/4 cup cooked (1 1/2 cup dry) black beans
1 tablespoon tomato paste

Toppings
Fat-free sour cream
Chopped cilantro
Diced tomato
Fat-free cheddar cheese

Directions
1. Heat oil in a large saucepan over medium heat.
2. Add onion, peppers, carrots and garlic to pan. Cook, stirring frequently, until onions are golden and veggies are tender (about 7 to 8 minutes).
3. Stir in chili powder and cumin. Cook 1 to 2 minutes.
4. Add ground turkey, stirring to break up the meat. Cook 5 to 7 minutes until meat is browned.
5. Transfer the meat and veggie mixture to a large soup pot. Add salsa, broth, beans, and tomato paste. Bring to a simmer over medium heat.
6. Lower the heat and simmer, uncovered, until the liquid has been reduced and the chili has thickened (about 45 to 50 minutes).
7. Check taste, adding spices if necessary. Serve with one or more toppings.

Makes 8 servings.

Troy Busot's Spinach Orzo Pasta Soup

Here's a quick and easy dinner idea for busy weeknights. You're just six ingredients away from "real fast food" that's nutritious and filling. This soup can be made vegetarian by using vegetable stock instead of chicken. If you want to add meat, try diced boneless, skinless chicken breast or Italian chicken sausage. As a time saver, I use chopped Italian tomatoes that have added oregano, basil, and garlic. If you have only plain canned tomatoes on hand, add one teaspoon each of dried oregano and basil and an additional clove of garlic.

Ingredients

Olive oil
1 large onion, chopped
2 cloves garlic, chopped
1 (15-ounce) can diced Italian tomatoes (with oregano and basil)
1 pound spinach
2 quarts chicken or vegetable stock
2 quarts water
1 pound orzo

Directions

1. In a large soup pot, heat olive oil. Add onions and saute until tender. Add garlic and saute 2 to 3 minutes. Add tomatoes, spinach, stock, and water. Bring to a boil. Reduce heat to medium.
2. Add orzo and cook 12 to 15 minutes, or until orzo is tender. Serve.

Makes 4 servings.

Troy Busot is the founder of Athlinks.com, which allows members of the endurance community to share their passion for competition and use that passion to grow the sport and make it accessible to athletes of all levels.

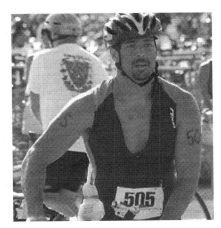

Photo courtesy of Troy Busot

Robin Thurston's Beet Juice Drink

Three simple ingredients—beets, apples, and carrots—don't sound like much, but sometimes the simple things give you the most bang for your buck. I have this quick-and-easy drink before every workout. You'll need a good juicer to properly prepare this recipe.

Ingredients
3 fresh beets
1 apple
3 carrots

Directions
Add each ingredient to the juicer and let the juicer do its magic. Pour into a glass and enjoy!

Robin Thurston is the cofounder and chief product officer of the MapMyFitness empire, which includes the popular websites MapMyRun.com, MapMyRide.com, and MapMyHike.com. The sites have more than 13 million registered members worldwide

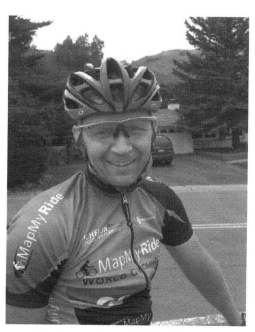

Photo courtesy of Robin Thurston

Toby Guillette's Apple Pie Oatmeal

This recipe is my go-to breakfast before long runs. It takes less than five minutes to make and is easy to eat first thing in the morning because of its comfort-food taste.

Ingredients

1 cup water
1 packet gluten-free oatmeal (Look for ingredients like gluten-free oats, raisins, maple sugar, brown sugar, flax meal, salt.)
1/2 apple, finely chopped
1 teaspoon cinnamon
1/2 teaspoon honey

Directions

1. In a small saucepan, bring water to a boil.
2. In a bowl, empty the packet of oatmeal. Add the apple.
3. Add enough boiling water to just cover the oatmeal and apple. Mix with spoon. Add cinnamon and honey and mix again. If consistency is too thick, add a bit more water and stir.

Makes 1 serving.

Toby Guillette is an ultra-endurance athlete, outdoor-adventure blogger and host of EnduranceGuy.com, and social media expert at the Active Network.

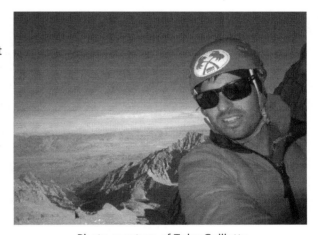

Photo courtesy of Toby Guillette

Judy Staveley's Chive Spread and Avocado Salad Sandwich

This sandwich incorporates a healthy bread that's awesome to keep on hand for sandwiches, toast, or just eating by itself.

Marathon Bread Ingredients
1 5/8 cups water
2 tablespoons honey
1 tablespoon molasses
1/4 cup shredded carrots
1/4 cup applesauce
2 1/2 cups bread flour
3/4 cup rye flour
3/4 cup white whole-wheat flour
1/3 cup flaxseed (half ground, half whole seed)
1/3 cup sunflower seeds
1/3 cup pumpkin seeds
2 tablespoons wheat germ
2 tablespoons rolled oats
2 tablespoons sesame seeds
2 tablespoons lecithin
2 tablespoons banana chips, chopped
1 tablespoon wheat gluten
1 teaspoon diastolic malt powder
1/2 teaspoon salt
1/8 teaspoon ascorbic acid
1 1/2 teaspoon instant yeast

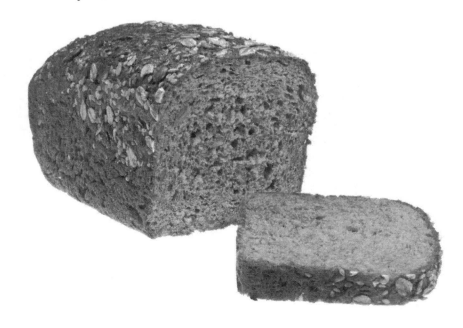

Avocado Salad Ingredients

1 avocado, peeled, pitted, and diced
1 tomato, cored and chopped
1 cucumber, peeled, seeded, and diced
Squeeze of lime juice
2 tablespoons chopped fresh basil or cilantro
Salt and pepper to taste

Chive Spread Ingredients

1/4 cup Greek yogurt
1 tablespoon finely chopped fresh chives
Salt and pepper to taste

Sandwich Ingredients

4 slices whole-grain bread (see Marathon Bread recipe in this section)
1/4 cup alfalfa sprouts
2 to 4 slices light pepper jack cheese

Bread Directions

Combine all ingredients in bread machine pan. Use the dough cycle only. Remove dough and shape into loaf. Place in greased 9-by-5-inch pan. Let rise until doubled, about 40 minutes. Bake at 375 degrees Fahrenheit for 40 to 45 minutes. Remove from pan and cool.

Avocado Salad, Chive Spread, and Sandwich Directions

1. In a medium bowl, gently toss together the avocado, tomato, cucumber, lime juice, and basil or cilantro. Season with salt and pepper. Set aside.
2. In a small bowl, mix the Greek yogurt and chives. Season with salt and pepper. Set aside.
3. Spread the chive-yogurt mixture on four bread slices. Divide the sprouts between two bread slices and top with avocado salad and cheese. Cover with the remaining bread slices.

Makes 2 large sandwiches.

Judy Staveley's Banana Oatmeal Smoothie

I love this easy-to-make recipe because it makes about 20 ounces of smoothie and provides about 28 grams of protein.

Ingredients
2 organic bananas
2 cups ice
1/2 cup cooked oatmeal
2 teaspoons flaxseed
1 scoop Hammer Protein
1/3 cup organic unsalted almonds
1/3 cup Greek yogurt

Directions
Combine all ingredients in a blender until smooth. Enjoy!

Judy Staveley is a professor and triathlete who teaches at colleges in the Maryland area. She's also CEO of *The Platform Magazine*. She serves as a spokeswoman and advocate for biological, health medicine, and forensic science organizations. Additionally, as a triathlete and national health and fitness specialist, she assists in community programs to initiate health in youth sports and is part of the USA swimming, USA hockey, and USAT organizations.

Staveley has been featured in presentations, media articles, and television appearances. While working as a professor, she remains active in her athletic and charitable pursuits and raises money for cancer, autism, and many other nonprofit organizations to help support families.

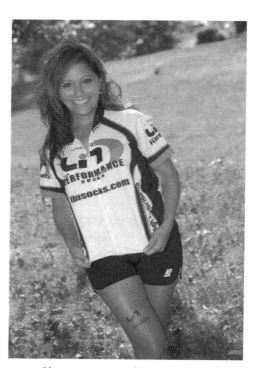

Photo courtesy of Judy Staveley

Ben Greenfield's High-Fat Smoothie

My breakfast of choice 99 percent of the time. Use a powerful blender for this one.

Ingredients
Handful of almonds
Handful of chia seeds
3 to 5 raw Brazil nuts
1/2 or whole avocado
1 teaspoon cinnamon
1 to 2 tablespoons cacao or carob powder
1 to 2 heaping scoops grass-fed whey or vegan protein power
4 to 6 ounces full-fat coconut milk (preferably a BPA-free variety)
Unsweetened coconut flakes or organic dark cacao nibs (optional)

Directions
In a blender, puree all ingredients until smooth. For a little crunch, add unsweetened coconut flakes or organic dark cacao nibs. Serve immediately. Makes 1 serving.

Ben Greenfield's Power Juice

This low-sugar power juice packs a punch of vitamins and digestive enzymes.

Ingredients
8 to 10 carrots
Chunk of ginger (about the size of a golf ball)
1 to 2 lemons
Small bunch of cilantro
1 to 2 teaspoons Himalayan salt
1 to 2 tablespoons extra-virgin olive oil
Ice

Directions
Add carrots, ginger, lemons, and cilantro to the juicer. Once the juice is made, stir in Himalayan salt and olive oil. Serve over ice. Makes 1 serving.

Ben Greenfield is a coach, author, speaker, ex-bodybuilder, and Ironman triathlete. Ben has revolutionized the way thousands of athletes and exercise enthusiasts around the world live, train, and eat. Ben works with athletes, CEOs, and soccer moms to achieve amazing feats of physical endurance without destroying their body in the process. Learn more at BenGreenfieldFitness.com.

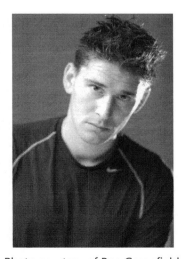

Photo courtesy of Ben Greenfield

Kenny Santucci's Banana and Egg Pancakes

This recipe sounds a bit odd, but as the old saying goes: Don't judge a book by its cover, or in this case, a recipe by its name. This simple dish requires only a few ingredients, cooks up in minutes, packs a punch of potassium and protein, and, best of all, tastes awesome! It's perfect before or after your workout.

Ingredients
1 banana
1/2 to 1 teaspoon cinnamon
Splash of vanilla
Dash of nutmeg
2 eggs

Directions
In a medium bowl, mash the banana. Add the cinnamon and mix well. Add vanilla and nutmeg and mix well. Add the eggs and mix well.

Heat pan or griddle to medium-high. With a ladle, pour the batter onto the griddle. Unlike traditional pancakes, these will not bubble on top to signal readiness to flip. Use a spatula to lift up the pancake edge to check for when it's ready to flip. Makes 2 to 3 pancakes.

Kenny Santucci wears many hats. You may recognize him as a reality star from MTV's *Challenge* series. Kenny has been a staple in many of the show's versions, most recently *Challenge Mania: The Road to Rivals II*. In addition to being a TV personality, he's an Ironman, triathlete, marathoner, adventure racer, college wrestler, Team ZICO member, a National Academy of Sports Medicine–certified personal trainer, a personal trainer at Equinox in New York City, and a motivational speaker.

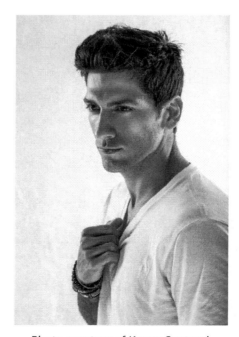

Photo courtesy of Kenny Santucci

Chef Brandon McDearis's Homemade Energy Gel

Chef Brandon McDearis was curious about what went into the energy gels that athletes use during training and racing events. He knew the ingredients were composed of simple carbs and some electrolytes, but the exact composition was a mystery. He was displeased with some of the ingredients he found in many gels, such as preservatives, natural flavors, pectin, xanthan gum, and gellan. So Brandon decided to create this recipe for a healthier, tastier homemade energy gel.

Ingredients
2 tablespoons chia seeds
2 tablespoons honey or agave
1 tablespoon brown rice or maple syrup
2 to 3 tablespoons water, salted with sea salt
1/4 teaspoon finely ground coffee
1/2 teaspoon cocoa
1 (3-ounce) travel shampoo bottle

Directions
1. In a medium bowl, mix chia seeds with salted water. Let them hydrate for a few minutes until they puff up and feel like they could almost be formed into a ball.
2. Add remaining ingredients and mix well. (Tip: For a more consistent coffee flavor, mix the coffee with 1 tablespoon of the water before combining it with the chia seeds. However, the stronger hints of ground coffee within the gel are also pleasant.)

The recipe yields about 3 to 4 ounces, enough to fill one 3-ounce travel shampoo bottle with a little bit left over. I find that the best way to get the mix from the bowl to the bottle is with a funnel. Small 1- to 2-ounce zip-close bags work great for storing the gel, especially the leftover ounce (or two) from the recipe.

Makes 3 to 4 servings. One-third of your bottle is the ideal shot of energy during times of exertion.

Chef Brandon McDearis's Breakfast Bowl

Is breakfast the most important meal of the day? Some argue that common claim, but physiology supports it. When you wake up, the body needs fuel because glycogen stores are low. The right breakfast gives you a mental advantage, plus insurance against fatigue, hunger, and overeating the wrong foods by lunchtime.

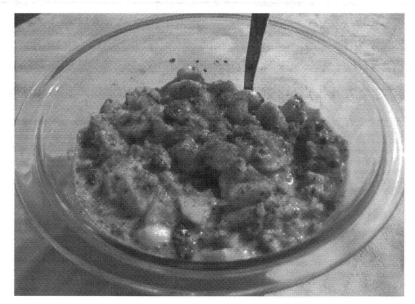

Photo courtesy of Brandon McDearis

This recipe is quick, easy, and loaded with nutrients that everyone should consume first thing in the morning. It's high in fiber and protein and low on the glycemic index, providing the mental and physical boost that we all need.

Ingredients
1/4 cup oats
1/4 cup water
1/4 small apple, diced
1/4 teaspoon cinnamon
1/2 scoop vanilla whey protein powder
1 tablespoon chia seeds
1 tablespoon raisins
2 ounces plain almond milk
1/2 medium banana, sliced

Directions
1. Microwave: In a medium bowl, combine the first three ingredients and microwave for 2 minutes on high. Stovetop: In a medium saucepan, bring the first three ingredients to a boil. Reduce heat to low. Cover and simmer until most of the liquid is evaporated.
2. Add remaining ingredients and mix well. Add a splash more water or almond milk for a thinner consistency.

Chef Brandon McDearis's
Quinoa with Garlic Chickpeas and Wilted Spinach

Quinoa is an excellent vegetarian option with all of the complete essential amino acids found in animal products and the bonus of being a whole grain. Chickpeas are also high in fiber and protein and contain phytochemicals that act as antioxidants. The immune-boosting and detoxifying onion and garlic, healthy fat in the olive oil, and high nutrition value of the spinach make this recipe all the more nourishing.

Ingredients
1 cup royal quinoa
2 to 3 tablespoons olive oil
1 small to medium onion, diced
3 to 4 cloves garlic, minced
1 can organic chickpeas
1/4 cup white wine
Juice from half a lemon
1/8 teaspoon cayenne or Tabasco
Salt and pepper to taste
2 cups baby spinach, packed tightly

Directions
1. Cook quinoa according to package directions.
2. Meanwhile, on medium-high heat, saute onion in olive oil for about 2 minutes. Add garlic and continue sauteing until the onion is soft and translucent. Add chickpeas and white wine and reduce heat to medium-low. Simmer 5 to 8 minutes, stirring frequently.
3. Once most of the wine has evaporated, remove from heat. Add the quinoa, lemon juice, and cayenne (or Tabasco) to the chickpea mixture. Season well with salt and pepper.
4. Last, incorporate the baby spinach a handful at a time. Makes 4 servings.

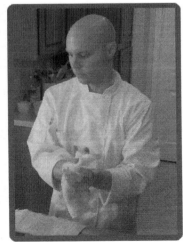

Brandon McDearis is a personal chef in Charlotte, North Carolina. In addition to his culinary training, Brandon holds a bachelor's degree in food and nutrition, with a concentration in dietetics. He focuses on healthy cooking and the dietary needs of everyone from professional and amateur athletes to busy families and senior citizens in his business, Your Way Cuisine (YourWayCuisine.com).

Brandon is a food and nutrition contributor for *Endurance Magazine*. He has also contributed to *Carolina Health and Fitness, US Rider News*, Livestrong.com, and *Whim Magazine*.

Photo courtesy of Brandon McDearis

Jason Robillard's Cheesy Hash Browns

One of my favorite snacks is a plate of hash browns topped with a sprinkling of cheese. This quick-and-easy dish is perfect before or after a run.

Ingredients
2 to 3 medium potatoes, peeled and grated (or 3 cups frozen shredded potatoes)
3 tablespoons olive oil
Salt and pepper to taste
1/2 cup shredded low-fat cheddar cheese

Directions
1. Arrange the grated potatoes between layers of paper towels. Press on the towels to absorb extra moisture from the potatoes.
2. In a saute pan on medium-high, heat the olive oil.
3. Arrange potatoes in the pan in an even layer. Add salt and pepper to taste.
4. Cook until bottom of potatoes is golden brown. (With a spatula, lift the edge to check doneness.) When the bottom is golden brown, flip the potato in one piece. If it breaks after flipping, simply piece it together in the pan.
5. Cook other side until golden brown.
6. Sprinkle with shredded cheese before removing from the pan. Cut the potato cake into fourths and serve.

Makes 4 servings.

Jason Robillard is the author of *The Barefoot Running Book*. Jason has also written articles for *Ultrarunning Magazine* and Competitor.com.

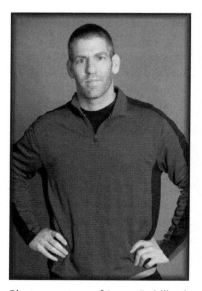

Photo courtesy of Jason Robillard

Chef Stefan Czapalay's Butternut Squash Soup

This recipe is so easy. Instead of squash, you can use carrots, parsnips, or sweet potatoes—or a combination of all three. When I return home from my long Sunday runs, in 60 seconds I have a cup of this steaming hot soup to sip on while stretching. It warms my core, and I can feel my body soaking in the vitamins. In summer I increase the orange juice to thin the soup a bit and drink it cold.

Ingredients
2 tablespoons olive oil
1 small onion, diced small
1 stalk celery, diced
1/2 teaspoon curry powder
1/4 teaspoon ground ginger
1 butternut squash, cut in large chunks
750 milliliters (about 3 cups) chicken stock
250 milliliters (about 1 cup) orange juice
1 bay leaf
Salt and pepper to taste
250 milliliters (about 1 cup) water, if needed

Directions
In a heavy-bottom saucepan, heat olive oil. Add onion, celery, curry powder, and ground ginger. Gently saute until aromatic, about 2 minutes. Add squash, chicken stock, orange juice, and bay leaf. Reduce heat to medium-low. Gently simmer for 30 minutes or until squash is tender. Adjust seasoning with salt and pepper. Puree with an immersion blender or mash with a whisk. If necessary, add water or chicken stock to thin to desired consistency.

Refrigerate soup if not eaten immediately. Reheat individual servings in a coffee mug in the microwave. Makes 12 servings.

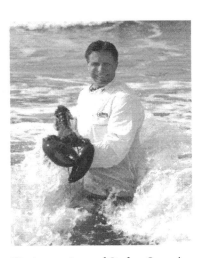

To define **Stefan Czapalay** as a chef is not as accurate as calling him a "culinary activist"—and he is among the best in Canada. Stefan is enthusiastic and passionate and has a constant hunger for innovation and learning. You'll find him at the helm of sustainable harvesting and wild-caught seafood movements, and working as corporate chef for Clearwater Seafoods, Canada's premier seafood supplier.

Photo courtesy of Stefan Czapalay

Kevin Leathers's Endurance Power Drink

This is my insurance to cover my nutritional blind spots and to fuel properly. I drink this every day for breakfast.

Ingredients

16 ounces water

1 scoop Green SuperFood by Amazing Grass (This gives me a full day's serving of fruits and vegetables, plus probiotics and enzymes to aid digestion. It's loaded with antioxidants and vitamins.)

1 scoop whey protein (Gives me 20 grams of protein to aid in muscle repair.)

2 tablespoons Udo's Oil 3-6-9 Blend (Aids in energy, recovery, and stamina. This is an organic, sustainable, fish-free blend of plant-sourced oils and contains all the good fats you need, without any of the bad fats you should avoid.)

Directions

Blend all ingredients until smooth. Drink immediately. Makes 1 serving.

Tip: To create a power recovery drink after long workouts or races, I add a scoop of GU Brew Recovery.

Kevin Leathers's Quick Oatmeal, Peanut Butter, and Fruit Breakfast

This is one of my favorite breakfast combos. It's a sturdy, filling meal for longer events that also makes a great recovery meal.

Ingredients

1 packet instant oatmeal

1/2 cup water

1 tablespoon peanut butter

1 banana, sliced or diced

Handful of blueberries

Directions

Prepare the oatmeal as directed on the package. Stir in the peanut butter and bananas, and top with blueberries. Makes 1 serving.

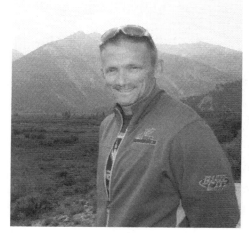

Photo courtesy of Kevin Leathers

Kevin Leathers is the host of the popular running blog CantStopEndurance.com. He's also an RRCA-certified running coach, national coach for the St. Jude Heroes program, national coach for the Team McGraw endurance program, and an accomplished runner, ultramarathoner, triathlete, and Ironman.

Laura Buxenbaum's Smoothie Recipes

Smoothies are a great way to get more nutrient-rich foods, such as fruit and dairy, into your diet. Use these recipes to get started, and experiment with your own favorite ingredients.

For each recipe, put the listed ingredients into a blender and blend at medium speed for two to three minutes or until it reaches your desired consistency.

Running Refuel Shake

1 cup fat-free chocolate milk

1 scoop 100% whey protein powder

1 banana

Crushed ice

Triple Berry Smoothie

1 cup low-fat vanilla yogurt

1 cup skim or 1% milk

1/3 cup frozen blueberries

1/3 cup frozen strawberries

1/3 cup frozen raspberries

Ice

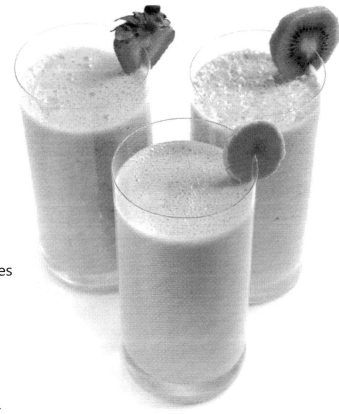

Orange Peach Mango Smoothie

1 cup orange juice

1 cup low-fat vanilla yogurt

1/2 cup frozen unsweetened peaches

1/2 cup frozen mangoes

Ice

PB&B Protein Smoothie

1 banana

1 tablespoon creamy peanut butter

1 cup 1% milk

1 scoop plain, vanilla, or chocolate whey protein powder

Crushed ice

Blues Buster Smoothie*

1 (6-ounce) container low-fat blueberry yogurt

1/2 cup apple juice

1/2 cup fresh or frozen blueberries

1/2 cup frozen sliced peaches

Crushed ice

*Recipe from SoutheastDairy.org

Benefits of Whey Protein

Whey protein is a high-quality, complete protein naturally found in dairy. It contains all of the essential amino acids your body needs to build and repair muscle. Whey protein is also an excellent source of branched-chain amino acids (BCAA), including leucine, which has been shown to stimulate muscle synthesis. Adding whey protein powder to smoothies enhances exercise recovery by helping build and repair muscle.

Laura Buxenbaum is a registered dietitian with more than 12 years of experience in clinical dietetics and nutrition education. She currently serves as the senior manager of nutrition affairs for the Southeast Dairy Association, where she is responsible for developing and conducting nutrition education programs for health professionals in North Carolina and Virginia.

Laura also works closely with the media to provide research-based nutrition information to the consumer through television, newspaper, and online interviews. She is an active member of the Academy of Nutrition and Dietetics and the Sports, Cardiovascular, and Wellness Nutrition Group. Laura is an avid exerciser who enjoys running, yoga, and hikes with her family. She believes in the power of nutrition for fueling and rebuilding tired muscles.

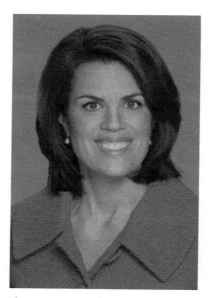

Photo courtesy of Laura Buxenbaum

More Running Fuel Recipes

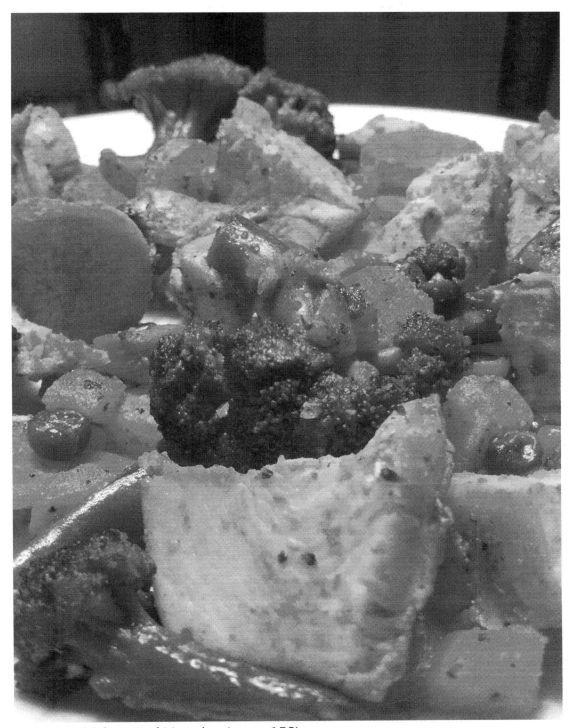

Healthy Chicken and Veggies (page 158)
Photo courtesy of Matthew Halip

Healthy Chicken and Veggies

This simple dish is similar to stir-fry but significantly healthier and lower in sodium. The original recipe came from Matthew Halip, a former lacrosse player for Guilford College and one of the exercise models for this book.

Ingredients
4 skinless, boneless chicken breasts
2 tablespoons olive oil
1 cup diced carrots
1 cup sweet corn
1 cup broccoli florets (Most any vegetable combination will work.)

Chicken Coating
In a medium bowl, combine these ingredients:
2 tablespoons chili powder
1/2 teaspoon ground white pepper
1/4 teaspoon allspice
Dash of salt
3 to 4 garlic cloves, minced
1 medium onion, chopped

Vinaigrette
2/3 cup olive oil
1/3 cup balsamic vinegar
2 teaspoons honey
1 tablespoon Dijon mustard

Mix olive oil, vinegar, honey, and mustard. The rule of thumb is two parts olive oil to one part vinegar, but you can change the ratio depending on your preference.

Directions
Preheat oven to 350 degrees Fahrenheit. Rub chicken with coating and place in a baking dish. Bake 15 to 20 minutes or until internal temperature reaches 165 degrees Fahrenheit. Let chicken rest for 5 minutes, and then cut into cubes.

Meanwhile, in a large frying pan on medium heat, drizzle vegetables with oil and stir-fry for 10 minutes. Mix cubed chicken into the vegetables. Pour vinaigrette over the mixture and cook for no more than 2 minutes. Once the chicken absorbs the marinade, remove from heat and serve. Makes 4 servings. (See photo of dish on page 157.)

Rotisserie Chicken Chili

One of my runners, Andy Manry, is quite the chef. He shared this chili recipe that has become a family favorite and makes a delicious recovery meal, particularly after a cold winter run. His dad turned him on to this dish, which Andy believes is based on a *Southern Living* recipe. You can find more of Andy's recipes at his blog, WhatsAndyCooking.blogspot.com.

Ingredients
2 tablespoons olive oil
1 red onion, chopped
3 cloves garlic, minced
1 red bell pepper, chopped
2 poblano peppers, seeded and chopped
2 (14-ounce) cans chili spiced tomatoes
2 (12-ounce) bottles of beer (Andy prefers an IPA, or you can use chicken stock.)
1 can navy beans
1 can black beans
1 packet McCormick's White Chicken Chili Mix
Meat from 1 rotisserie chicken (or 1 smoked chicken), shredded

Directions
In a large heavy pot over medium-high, heat olive oil until shimmering. Add onion, garlic, bell pepper, and poblano peppers and saute until onions are translucent, stirring often. You want the veggies to sweat like you did during your run.

Add tomatoes, beer (or stock), navy and black beans, chili mix, and chicken. Bring to a boil. Reduce heat to low and simmer 1 hour or more, until you're ready to eat. If simmering for more than 1 hour, cover the pot after 30 minutes.

Serve with your favorite chili toppings or enjoy it plain. My favorite topping is a mix of roasted corn, lime, and cilantro. To cook this, add 1 tablespoon olive oil to a nonstick pan over medium-high heat. Add 2 cups frozen corn and cook just until the corn begins to blacken. Sprinkle with a little chili powder, cumin, chopped fresh cilantro, salt, and pepper. Squeeze the juice of 2 limes into the corn mixture, stir, and remove from heat. Other popular toppings include chopped green onions, sour cream, and cheese. Enjoy!

Gabby's Vegetarian Chili

Gabriela Huynh, a runner friend from Silicon Valley, California, sent me this veggie chili recipe that has become a staple in my training nutrition. There are a lot of ingredients, but the final product is worth it. This dish will feed a family with plenty of leftovers. It tastes even better the next day and is full of protein and carbs, perfect to eat after a long run or hard track workout.

Ingredients

2 (28-ounce) cans diced tomatoes
4 cups (roughly 2 cans) reduced-sodium vegetable broth
1 (15-ounce) can black beans, rinsed and drained
1 (15-ounce) can white beans, rinsed and drained
1 (15-ounce) can kidney beans, rinsed and drained
1 cup chopped onion
1 green bell pepper
2 cloves garlic, minced (or 1 tablespoon garlic powder)
1 tablespoon (or 1 whole) minced jalapeno, fresh or canned
1 packet chili seasoning (also works with taco or burrito seasoning)
2 tablespoons Mexican oregano
2 tablespoons ground cumin
4 to 5 dashes hot sauce (optional)
Salt and pepper to taste
1/2 pound macaroni (or 1/3 cup couscous)
1/2 cup shredded Jack cheese (optional)
1/3 cup chopped cilantro

Directions

In a slow cooker, combine all ingredients except pasta, cilantro, and shredded cheese. Cover and cook on low 6 to 8 hours or on high 3 to 4 hours. Cook pasta to desired texture and add to slow cooker 10 minutes before serving. Serve topped with cheese and cilantro.

Quick & Easy Chicken Primavera

This meal is versatile and simple, requiring just grilled chicken tenderloins, pasta, frozen veggies, and a few spices. Multigrain pasta is your best choice, but have fun and mix it up. Try 100 percent whole wheat or tricolor pasta, as well as different shapes, such as rotini, penne, fettuccine, or angel hair. Protein-rich chickpeas and chicken make this dish a perfect post-run meal. It also keeps well in the fridge, so make extra to enjoy for lunch the rest of the week.

Ingredients
1 box multigrain or tricolor pasta of your choice
2 tablespoons olive oil
6 boneless, skinless chicken breast tenderloins
1 can chickpeas (aka garbanzo beans), rinsed and drained
1 package frozen mixed vegetables (such as broccoli, cauliflower, and carrots)
1 medium onion, chopped
Lawry's Seasoning Salt to taste
Grated Parmesan cheese

Directions
Cook pasta according to package directions. In a large skillet, heat olive oil and chopped onion over medium heat. While onions are cooking, in a well-oiled skillet, cook chicken tenderloins 2 to 3 minutes each side or until lightly browned. Cut into bite-size chunks. When onions are translucent, add the chickpeas. Steam the vegetables. Drain the pasta, add a little olive oil, and stir. Add pasta to the onion and chickpea mixture, then add chicken and veggies. Add seasoning salt to taste (it doesn't take much). Stir until combined. Serve topped with Parmesan cheese.

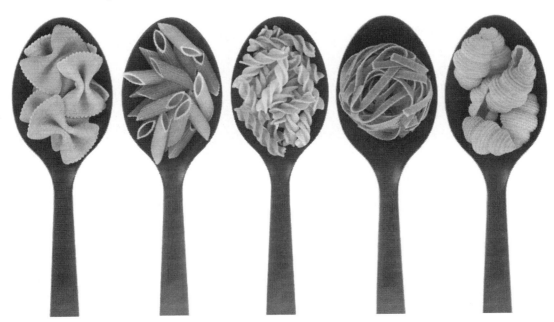

Rice and Bean Burritos

You'll be amazed how easy these burritos are to make. They're also high in protein and low in fat—perfect for after training or to pack for lunch. My kids love 'em!

Ingredients
1 1/2 cups instant brown rice (uncooked)
1 tablespoon olive oil
1/2 cup chopped onion
1 medium green pepper
1 tablespoon chili powder
1 teaspoon ground cumin
1/8 teaspoon crushed red pepper flakes (optional)
1 (15-ounce) can black beans, rinsed and drained
1 (15-ounce) can corn, rinsed and drained
8 whole-wheat tortillas
1 cup salsa
Reduced-fat shredded Mexican-blend cheese
Reduced-fat sour cream

Directions
Prepare rice according to package directions. Meanwhile, in a large skillet, heat olive oil. Saute onion and green pepper until tender (just a few minutes). Add chili powder, cumin, and red pepper flakes. Stir until well combined. Add beans, corn, and cooked rice to the pan and cook for 5 minutes, stirring constantly. Wrap stacked tortillas in a paper towel and warm in the microwave for about 1 minute. Spoon rice and bean mixture onto the center of each tortilla. If desired, top with salsa, cheese, and sour cream. Fold the sides of each tortilla over and roll up like a burrito. Makes 8 burritos.

Variations
- Instead of black beans, try pinto, kidney, or navy or use a mixture.
- Want more protein? Add diced grilled chicken breast.
- No time to cook beans and rice? Use canned fat-free refried beans instead. Simply spoon the desired amount onto a tortilla and heat it in the microwave for about 30 seconds. Add your toppings and wrap.

Quinoa Chicken with Vegetables

The quinoa in this dish is a great alternative to pasta. An "ancient grain" (technically the seed of the goosefoot plant), quinoa is a power food that provides all of the essential amino acids, making it a complete protein.

Ingredients
1 tablespoon olive oil
2 skinless, boneless chicken breast halves
1 cup uncooked red or white quinoa
2 cups low-sodium vegetable broth
2 (12-ounce) packages frozen mixed vegetables (steamed are a healthy choice)
Salt to taste

Directions
1. Coat a large skillet with olive oil and heat over medium-high. Add chicken breasts and cook for 1 minute. Flip and cook for another minute. Cover, reduce heat to medium-low, and cook 6 to 9 minutes, flipping chicken frequently. When done, remove chicken from pan and cut into chunks.
2. While the chicken is cooking, prepare the quinoa. In a saucepan, combine quinoa and broth and bring to a boil. Reduce to a simmer, cover, and cook 10 to 15 minutes.
3. While the quinoa is cooking, prepare frozen vegetables according to package directions.
4. In a large bowl, combine chicken, quinoa, and vegetables. Salt to taste, if desired.

Makes 4 servings.

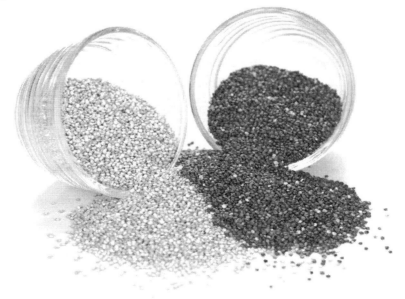

Healthy Pancakes on the Run

I was late to meet my buddies for a long run and didn't have time for my usual breakfast, so I grabbed what was handy: a leftover pancake. I folded it over like a taco and ate it cold with no syrup. Delicious—and I felt great during my run!

That batch was from a box mix. I tried to create a healthier version using regular whole-wheat flour, but they were too heavy. That flour is made from red wheat, which has a coarse texture and slightly bitter taste. I decided to give unbleached white whole-wheat flour a try. This flour is made from an albino wheat that has a smoother texture and sweeter taste, yet provides the same health benefits as the regular variety and is not bleached or bromated. The result is a lighter, milder-tasting pancake. Enjoy!

Ingredients
2 cups 100% unbleached white whole-wheat flour, sifted
2 teaspoons baking powder
1 scoop vanilla-flavored whey protein powder
4 egg whites (Liquid egg whites also work well.)
1 1/2 cups skim milk
3 tablespoons canola oil
2 tablespoons honey
2 teaspoons vanilla or butternut flavoring

Directions
In a large bowl, combine dry ingredients. In a separate bowl, combine liquid ingredients. Add liquid mixture to dry ingredients and stir until combined (a few lumps are okay). Preheat a nonstick griddle to 375 degrees Fahrenheit. Ladle batter onto griddle and cook both sides until golden. Makes eight 5-inch pancakes.

Variations
- Make a double batch and store leftovers in zipper bags. Reheat on a plate in the microwave for 30 to 35 seconds.
- Want less oil? Substitute applesauce or another egg white for some of the oil.
- Fewer calories? Use Splenda instead of honey.
- More texture and protein? Add pecans or walnuts to the batter.
- More sweetness? Add blueberries, strawberries, or bananas to the batter.

Throw-It-in-a-Pot Chicken and Pasta Surprise

If you like recipes that are quick, easy, and healthy, then you'll love this dish. Full of energy-providing complex carbohydrates and muscle-rebuilding protein, it's ideal after a long run.

Ingredients

2 precooked chicken breasts
12 ounces multigrain pasta
1 can diced tomatoes (do not drain liquid)
1 medium onion, chopped
4 cloves garlic, sliced
1/2 teaspoon red pepper flakes
2 teaspoons dried oregano
2 sprigs basil, chopped
4 1/2 cups vegetable broth
2 tablespoons extra-virgin olive oil
Parmesan cheese

Directions

1. Place the chicken breasts on a microwave-safe plate. Cover with a paper towel. Microwave on high for 3 1/2 to 4 minutes.
2. While the chicken is heating, in a large pot, combine the pasta, tomatoes, onion, garlic, red pepper flakes, oregano, and basil. Add broth and pour olive oil over the top of the mixture. Cover and bring to a boil. Once boiling, reduce heat to low and simmer about 10 minutes or until most of the liquid has evaporated, stirring every couple of minutes. Salt and pepper to taste, and stir mixture well.
3. Plate the pasta and top with Parmesan cheese, if desired.

Makes 5 servings.

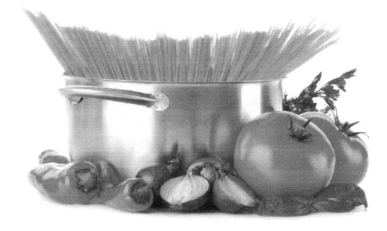

RunnerDude's Pumpkin Smoothie

Pumpkins are often thought of as a seasonal holiday food, but they're also an excellent source of potassium and vitamin A, making this simple smoothie ideal for before or after your run.

Ingredients

1/2 cup pumpkin puree
1/2 cup fat-free vanilla Greek yogurt
1 banana, sliced into chunks
1 teaspoon pumpkin pie spice
1/2 cup skim milk
1 teaspoon vanilla extract
1 cup ice

Directions

Add all ingredients to a blender container and blend for 2 to 3 minutes. For a thinner consistency, add another 1/2 cup skim milk. For extra sweetness, add 1 tablespoon honey.

Makes about 2 1/2 cups.

Breakfast Burrito

Fellow runner and friend Jeff Pickett shared this delicious recipe for a simple breakfast or anytime meal that's perfect before or after your run. You'll be amazed how easy these burritos are to make. They're also high in protein and low in fat.

Ingredients
Cooking spray
4 egg whites
1 whole egg
2 tortillas
Light sour cream
Fat-free or reduced-fat shredded cheddar cheese
Salsa

Directions:
1. Spray a nonstick frying pan with cooking spray.
2. Combine egg whites and whole egg in the pan. Cook eggs for a few minutes until it forms an omelet. Flip and cook the other side.
3. Heat tortillas in the microwave for 8 to 10 seconds. Place tortillas on separate plates. Spread a thin layer of sour cream over each tortilla.
4. Cut the omelet in half and place one half onto each tortilla so that half of the tortilla is covered with the omelet. Sprinkle each omelet half with shredded cheddar cheese. Top with salsa. Fold tortillas over filling and enjoy!

Makes 2 burritos.

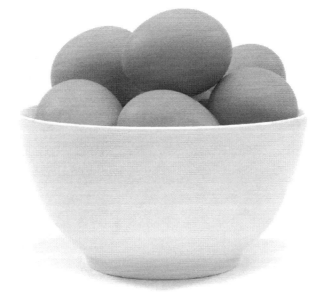

About the Author

Thad McLaurin has come a long way since being "that overweight kid" who ran an 18-minute mile in plaid pants and Wallabees in the eighth grade. That summer he began a weight-loss quest and lost 40 pounds before beginning high school. He discovered his love of running in college when running his very first race—the Great Raleigh Road Race 10K. He wasn't fast, but he had a blast and was hooked. Thad's been passionate about running and fitness ever since (30 years!).

A UNC-Chapel Hill grad, Thad began his professional life as a fifth-grade teacher before moving on to educational publishing, where he worked as a writer, editor, and book development manager for 13 years. Thad continues to combine his love of writing with his love of running and fitness by hosting the popular website RunnerDude's Blog (RunnerDudesBlog.com), one of the top-ranked running blogs in the country. He's also a contributing writer for Active.com, has written articles for AmateurEndurance.com, and was featured in the July 2010 *Runner's World* "Ask the Experts" section.

During the economic crash, in 2009, Thad was laid off from his position at the publishing company. A bit lost and unsure where to turn next, he decided to pursue his passion—running and fitness. Both excited and nervous, he returned to school and earned his diploma from the National Personal Training Institute. Thad is also an ACSM certified personal trainer and an RRCA and USA Track and Field certified running coach.

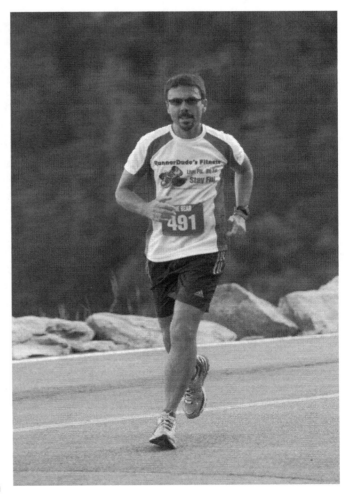

In 2010, Thad opened RunnerDude's Fitness, a personal training studio in Greensboro, North Carolina, that provides fitness and running programs for all ages and ability levels. He has worked with hundreds of runners, from beginners to experienced marathoners. His biggest reward is helping others get hooked on running, fitness, and healthy living.

Thad, his wife, Mitzi, and their three kids—Duncan, Rayna, and Ellery—live in Greensboro, North Carolina.

TRUST in your training,
BELIEVE in yourself, and you'll
CONQUER your goals!

—RunnerDude

Made in the USA
Lexington, KY
05 March 2017